**"This book is a peek inside the minds of clinical scientists who are doing cutting-edge research on attachment, compassion, shame, parenting, mindfulness, and positive psychology. The content offered on this cluster of topics is thoroughly satisfying while it inspires readers to pursue their own informed questions. Highly recommended for curious clinicians of all stripes – students, academics, and professionals."**

– Christopher Germer, PhD, Harvard Medical School, USA

**"Compassion-focussed psychotherapy is the most promising treatment for emotion disorders that have not responded well to other therapies. This is simply the best introduction to this extraordinarily valuable approach. It is highly recommended for experienced practitioners, as well as those starting out in psychotherapeutic practice."**

– Professor Peter Fonagy OBE, Head of Division for Psychology and Language Sciences at UCL, UK

**"Packed with cutting-edge research, clinical wisdom and a satisfying mixture of compassionate commitment and serious scholarship, this book is a major contribution to understanding psychological wellbeing. It is a treat of a book written by experts who care for their subject deeply, and will be of great help to researchers, mental health professionals, students and many more."**

– Graham Music, PhD, Tavistock Clinic London, UK, and author of *Nurturing Children* and *Nurturing Natures*

# MAKING AN IMPACT ON MENTAL HEALTH

Advancements in research in psychological science have afforded great insights into how our minds work. *Making an Impact on Mental Health* analyses contemporary, international research to examine a number of core themes in mental health, such as mindfulness and attachment, and provides an understanding of the sources of mental ill health and strategies for remediation.

The originality of this work is the embedding of psychological science in an evolutionary approach. Each chapter discusses the context of a specific research project, looking at the methodological and practical challenges, how the results have been interpreted and communicated, the impact and legacy of the research and the lessons learnt. As a whole, the book looks at how social environments shape who we are and how we form relationships with others, which can be detrimental, but equally a source of flourishing and well-being.

Covering a range of themes conducive to understanding and facilitating improved mental health, *Making an Impact on Mental Health* is invaluable reading for advanced students in clinical psychology and professionals in the mental health field.

**James N. Kirby** is Senior Lecturer and Clinical Psychologist at the University of Queensland, Australia. He examines how compassion can help create nurturing family environments.

**Paul Gilbert** is world-renowned for his work on compassion, depression, shame and self-criticism. He received an OBE for his contributions to mental health.

## Routledge Psychological Impacts

Series Editor: Graham Davey

*Routledge Psychological Impacts* is a series of books illustrating how psychological research can make meaningful contributions to social policy. Each book in the series covers a specific topic, showcasing a range of research projects that have either made a direct impact on policy, or brought about a wider awareness of the issues.

Chapters in the books describe the context of specific research projects, discuss the methodological and practical challenges faced by the researchers, and describe how the results are interpreted and communicated before outlining the impact and legacy of the research. Within each chapter, contributors discuss what lessons they learnt in the process, as well as offering advice to the research community about engaging with policy issues.

With the understanding of human behaviour as one of the main purposes of psychological science, psychological research has a great deal to contribute when it comes to finding solutions for our important social problems. This series aims to describe how psychologists are making a difference.

**Making an Impact on School Bullying**
*Edited by Peter K. Smith*

**Making an Impact on Mental Health**
*Edited by James N. Kirby and Paul Gilbert*

For more information about this series, please visit: www.routledge.com/Routledge-Pschological-Impacts/book-series/IMPACTS

# MAKING AN IMPACT ON MENTAL HEALTH

## The Applications of Psychological Research

*Edited by James N. Kirby and Paul Gilbert*

Routledge
Taylor & Francis Group
LONDON AND NEW YORK

First published 2021
by Routledge
2 Park Square, Milton Park, Abingdon, Oxon OX14 4RN

and by Routledge
52 Vanderbilt Avenue, New York, NY 10017

*Routledge is an imprint of the Taylor & Francis Group, an informa business*



*British Library Cataloguing-in-Publication Data*
A catalogue record for this book is available from the British Library

*Library of Congress Cataloging-in-Publication Data*
A catalog record for this book has been requested

ISBN: 978-0-367-19989-0 (hbk)
ISBN: 978-0-367-19990-6 (pbk)
ISBN: 978-0-429-24455-1 (ebk)

Typeset in Bembo
by Apex CoVantage, LLC

# CONTENTS

# CONTRIBUTORS

**Ernst T. Bohlmeijer** is Professor of Mental Health Promotion at the University of Twente in the Netherlands. His research focuses on promoting mental well-being, establishing the scientific foundation of sustainable mental health and evaluating the impact of interventions that promote sustainable mental health. He has a special interest in positive psychology, compassion-based interventions, acceptance and commitment therapy and life-review. He is author of the self-help book *Using Positive Psychology Every Day* that is increasingly used in mental health care as part of well-being therapy.

**Graham Davey** is Professor of Psychology at University of Sussex, UK. He is the Series Editor for *Routledge Psychological Impacts*. His research interests extend across mental health problems, generally, and anxiety and worry, specifically.

**Paul Gilbert** is world-renowned for his work on compassion, depression, shame and self-criticism. He received an OBE for his contributions to mental health and is author of *The Compassionate Mind* and *Overcoming Depression*.

**Felicia Huppert** specialises in the science of well-being and the promotion of human flourishing. Her current research focuses on mindfulness and compassion training in education and healthcare, and high-quality measures of subjective well-being. Felicia is Visiting Professorial Fellow at the University of New South Wales in Sydney, Australia, and spends part of the year in the UK, where she is Founding Director of the Well-being Institute at the University of Cambridge and Emeritus Professor of Psychology. She is a member of the Australian Expert Group of the Global Mindfulness Initiative and Director of the Australian Compassion Council Scholars Program.

**James N. Kirby** is Senior Lecturer, Clinical Psychologist and Co-Director of the Compassionate Mind Research Group at the University of Queensland, Australia. James' research has examined the impact of compassion focused approaches on mental health and how compassion can help cultivate nurturing family environments. He has published over 60 peer-reviewed publications that have examined compassion, family and mental health. He continues to work as a clinical psychologist helping individuals with self-criticism and shame.

**Geoff MacDonald** is Professor of Psychology at the University of Toronto, Canada, whose research interests include adult attachment, intimacy, sexuality and singlehood.

**Marcela Matos** is Clinical Psychologist and Researcher Faculty member at the Center for Research in Neuropsychology and Cognitive and Behavioral Interventions (CINEICC), University of Coimbra, Portugal. For 15 years, Dr. Matos' research and clinical interests have related to evolutionary clinical psychology, third-wave cognitive and behavioural therapies and contemplative approaches. She has extensively researched shame experiences and memories, their traumatic qualities and centrality to personal identity, and their association to mental health difficulties. Her current research involves developing, implementing and trialling compassion focused interventions for promoting well-being, and investigating their impact on epigenetic mechanisms and biophysiological markers of prosociality and stress.

**Christopher A. Pepping** is Senior Lecturer in Clinical Psychology at La Trobe University, Australia. His research interests include adult attachment, close relationships, singlehood and LGBTIQ mental health.

**José Pinto-Gouveia** is a psychiatrist, former Head of the Center for Research in Neuropsychology and Cognitive and Behavioral Interventions (CINEICC), and retired Full Professor, Faculty of Psychology and

Educational Sciences, University of Coimbra, Portugal. He has developed and led several research projects in third-wave cognitive and behavioural therapies. He is the co-founder of the Portuguese Association of Behavior Therapy and President of the Portuguese Association for Mindfulness. He has authored over 250 scientific papers, books and chapters in several physical and psychological conditions, namely psychological adjustment in cancer patients, chronic pain, infertility, obesity, anxiety, depression, personality disorders and eating disorders.

**Stan Steindl** is a clinical psychologist in private practice at Psychology Consultants Pty Ltd, and Adjunct Associate Professor at the School of Psychology, University of Queensland, Australia. He is also the co-director of the UQ Compassionate Mind Research Group. He has over 20 years' experience as a therapist, supervisor and trainer, and works clinically in the areas of shame, trauma and addiction. His research explores compassion and compassion-based interventions, and especially the role of cultivating compassion and self-compassion in the context of trauma, shame, self-criticism and clinical disorders, as well as promoting psychological well-being.

**Cassandra L. Tellegen**, PhD, is Senior Research Fellow and Clinical Psychologist at the School of Psychology at the University of Queensland, Australia. Cassandra's research has focused on how best to support parents of children who have autism. Her work examines the impact of family-based interventions to help support parents, children and families. Cassandra has published extensively in the field of clinical and family psychology. She continues to work as a clinical psychologist helping individuals with autism.

**Gerben J. Westerhof** is Professor of Narrative Psychology and Technology at the University of Twente in the Netherlands. His main research focus is how stories are related to mental health and well-being across the lifespan. He is interested in method development, like the use of computational methods in the verbal and nonverbal analysis of storytelling. He also developed and evaluated several (digital) narrative interventions to promote well-being in older adults and in people with psychiatric complaints.

**Nickolas Yu** is a qualified nurse, coach and meditation facilitator. He is a leader in workplace meditation and evidence-based healthcare coaching. He pioneered meditation-based wellness and compassion

(MWAC) training and evidence-based coaching in NSW Health, Australia. MWAC now has more than 7,000 attendees annually. Nickolas is skilled at making meditation principles and practices accessible to busy professionals within a science-informed, non-religious context. Nickolas is the Program Manager for Staff Wellness and Patient and Family-centred Care at Sydney Local Health District. He is a member of the Australian Compassion Council Scholars Program and Sydney University Body Heart and Mind in Business Research Group.

# SERIES FOREWORD

*Routledge Psychological Impacts* is a series of books illustrating how psychological research can make meaningful contributions to social policy. Each book in the series covers a specific topic, showcasing a range of research projects that have either made a direct impact on policy or brought about a wider awareness of the issues.

Chapters in the books describe the context of specific research projects, discuss the methodological and practical challenges faced by researchers, and describe how the results are interpreted and communicated before outlining the impact and legacy of the research. Within each chapter, contributors discuss what lessons they learnt in the process, as well as offer advice to the research community about engaging with policy issues.

In this volume on the impact of psychological research on mental health practice, editors James N. Kirby and Paul Gilbert have invited a number of international mental health researchers to reflect on how their research helps us to understand mental health problems, how we can develop effective interventions for these problems, and then how we might go about converting these successes into policies that are adopted for the benefit of everyone within our society.

The overriding theme of the book is that psychological science is becoming much more integrated and interdisciplinary, and psychology researchers are combining knowledge from many different areas to create effective interventions and therapies. In particular, the authors within this volume discuss the links between approaches such as evolutionary functional analysis and the importance of social relationships, and discuss how basic research is converted into effective intervention programs – sometimes successfully, but in other cases by having to confront a variety of obstacles before easy access to treatment for mental health problems can be provided.

Graham Davey

# INTRODUCTION TO PSYCHOLOGICAL IMPACTS ON MENTAL HEALTH

## How psychological science informs how we approach mental health

*James N. Kirby and Paul Gilbert*

We were delighted to be asked to edit this volume, inviting a selection of international researchers to reflect on how their area of research helps us understand and develop therapies for mental health problems. This volume is one in the series of volumes edited by Graham Davey for Routledge that invites researchers to reflect on their work in detail and contributions to their discipline. We thought it was a fascinating and new approach to exploring research on mental health difficulties.

There is increasing evidence that mental health is the result of a range of complex interacting processes. These include genes and their epigenetic regulation via social and ecological processes especially early in life. We also know that our 'brains' are more changeable than we thought 20 years ago. The understanding of neuroplasticity has meant that therapies are developing to target particular physiological systems. As discussed elsewhere research in mental health is becoming more consilient, interdisciplinary and integrative (Gilbert, 2019; Gilbert & Kirby, 2019). We have therefore invited authors to outline their specific areas of research and how they see it as adding to our greater understanding of the complexities and alleviation of mental health problems.

We begin with highlighting the importance of rooting psychological science in an evolutionary function analytic approach. As has often been said, 'Nothing makes sense in biology or indeed psychology in the absence of an evolutionary approach'. The evolutionary approach helps us understand the origins of motives, needs, emotions and cognitive competencies. The first chapter by Gilbert focuses on motivational systems underpinning social competition that give rise to issues and concerns with social position, social comparison, sense of inferiority, shame and vulnerability to depression.

Another major evolutionary process is of course attachment. We now know that the experiences we have in our early life have a range of long-term impacts even at the epigenetic level. Indeed it is our attachment experiences that can set the scene for us to become very orientated in the competitive dynamics of life and concerned with inferiority, self-criticism, and shame; attachment research is now a vast area of research. In Chapter 2 Pepping and MacDonald outline their own research program and how that has contributed to the attachment research history and insight into mental health problems.

Our third chapter looks at parenting. The early attachment contexts give rise to how children experience their families and parenting. The different styles of parenting therefore are very important for understanding the context in which children grow and mature. Again research into parenting styles and the impact on child maturation is a huge area of research. Here Kirby and Tellegen link evolutionary functional analysis to issues of attachment and their own studies of parenting styles and child impacts.

Chapter 4 considers some of the problems that can arise from difficult early childhoods. Clearly, there are many consequences to problematic attachment and parenting. One of them is our disposition to grow in an atmosphere of shame and being ashamed. There is good evidence that early experiences of shame predispose individuals to difficulties in social relationships, problems with trust, difficulties with emotion regulation and significantly increased vulnerability to mental health problems. Indeed, shame is probably one of the most common transdiagnostic processes underpinning mental health difficulties. Based on extensive research by Matos and colleagues, this chapter explores core issues on shame, in particular how shame memories are like trauma memories.

Chapter 5 addresses themes of recent innovations in psychotherapy. Again this is a huge area which has seen many impressive developments in the last 20 years. One of the most notable has been the way in which contemplative traditions have influenced therapeutic engagement. One of these is mindfulness. There are many concepts and definitions of mindfulness and how they have been integrated into mental health work. In this chapter Huppert and Yu explore their own approach and research into mindfulness and how it contributes to the wider research agenda on mindfulness and can be used therapeutically.

Last but not least, our sixth chapter focuses on a very important concept of flourishing. While it is true that we need to understand the causes and alleviation of mental health difficulties this in itself is not sufficient to help live prosocial and meaningful lives. The clinical sciences must also be concerned with what gives people meaning and helps them to flourish. Rooted in positive psychology, Bohlmeijer and Westerhof outline the research program on flourishing and how it can also contribute to creating conditions for mental well-being and offsetting problems in mental health difficulties.

No doubt different editors would have chosen different subject areas and different individuals because our science is so vast. However we hope that readers gain a sense of underlying themes with these chapters linking evolutionary functional analysis with the importance of social relationships as foundations for mental health. The idea is that each invited author would reflect on their own research and contribution. They explore their reasons for the research area and methodologies they have developed. We also hope that these insights into particular personal research programs will inspire others and give insights into research journeys.

## References

Gilbert, P. (2019). Psychotherapy for the 21st century: An integrative, evolutionary, contextual, biopsychosocial approach. *Psychology and Psychotherapy: Theory, Research and Practice, 92*, 164–189. doi:10.1111/papt.12226

Gilbert, P., & Kirby, J. N. (2019). Building an integrative science for psychotherapy for the 21st century: Preface and introduction. *Psychology and Psychotherapy: Theory, Research and Practice, 92*, 151–163. doi:10.1111/papt.12225

# 1

# EVOLUTIONARY FUNCTIONAL ANALYSIS

## The study of social mentalities, social rank and caring-compassion

*Paul Gilbert*

### The context of the research

The chapters of this book are designed to explore a focus on specific scientific approaches to mental health problems, noting their origins, development and implications for intervention. With that in mind this chapter offers a personal overview of my interest and research in evolutionary and social contextual approaches to mental health problems (Gilbert, 1984, 1989, 2019a). Special interest is given to social mentality theory that is focused on social motives, social cognition and reciprocal dynamic interpersonal behaviours associated with the co-creation of social roles (e.g., status, sexual, friendly, caring) (Gilbert, 1989, 1992, 2017a). It will outline the historical context for the research program of the last 40 years (Gilbert, 2007). I will be reviewing my own research program but not the substantial literature on evolutionary psychology and approaches to mental health problems (see Brüne, 2015; Dunbar, 2017; Dunbar & Barrett, 2007; McGuire & Troisi, 1998; Nesse, 2019; Sapolsky, 2017; Sloman & Gilbert, 2000).

#### *Personal journey*

My story begins with my first PhD studies in the 1970s at the University of Edinburgh on the psychological and physiological reactions of anxious and depressed people to success and failure events.

Using the galvanic skin response, I found that they respond similarly to failure events but depressed people under responded to success events supporting the idea that depression was linked to problems of positive affect and poor responses to rewards (Gilbert, 1980). What intrigued me then, and has for the rest of my research life, is why would such a mental state like depression, which seems so maladaptive, cause such misery and can end in suicide, be so prevalent in humans? The World Health Organisation (2018) estimates there are well over 300 million depressed people in the world today, and that suicide 'was the second leading cause of death among 15–29 year-olds'. In addition, many millions more suffer from sub-clinical syndromes and can find life hard and miserable. These questions began my first steps into what is called evolutionary functional analysis (EFA), the need to understand the evolved functional systems underpinning distressing mental states (Gilbert, 1984, 1992, 1989, 1998, 2019a; Buss, 2015).

Working at the Edinburgh Medical Research Council unit in the 1970s, which was doing considerable work in the psychopharmacology of depression, I was interested in exploring the psychosocial processes that might drive some of the physiological underpinnings, vulnerability, triggering, maintenance of and recovery from depression (Gilbert, 1988, 1995, 2013, 2016, 2019a); hence the title of my first book *Depression: From Psychology to Brain State* (Gilbert, 1984). It reviewed the literature on how psychological processes and social contexts could drive physiological ones such as reductions in dopamine and serotonin, elevate cortisol and knock out frontal cortical function. This book also looked at factors that produce discontinuities and non-linear changes in brain state patterns of activation, using what was then called catastrophe theory. The idea was to move away from the concept of fixed states, that change could be non-linear and discontinuous, and consider the ways in which mental states can move dynamically, and at times erratically, with sudden switches rather than smooth transitions. These can all be seen as 'normal functions' of a brain under certain types of contextual stress.

EFA was a steppingstone into a biopsychosocial approach (Gilbert, 1984, 1989, 1995, 2013). It offers a way of thinking about the origins and nature of physical and mental characteristics and asks questions like: why do we have (say) two legs, two arms, sensory faculties, a digestive tract, cardiovascular and immune systems; what is the value of a physical system that can vomit, have diarrhoea and raise temperature, which in certain contexts can also kill us (Nesse & Williams, 1995)? Psychological processes can also be viewed through an evolutionary lens in terms of their distal and proximal origins. So we can ask questions like: why do we have the set of emotions, motives and cognitive competencies that we do? How and why did they get built like that? What are they designed to do? How do they function? What are their underlying mechanisms? How are they regulated? How do different environments impact on their development and function? What do they need in order to function optimally? And of course, why can they be the source of so much mental pain and suffering? EFA today is now helping us understand the nature of many basic motives, emotions and competencies, including processes such as attachment, morality, sexuality, status seeking, affect regulation and competencies like empathy and our unique form of consciousness and conscious awareness (Bernard, Mills, Swenson, & Walsh, 2005; Crawford & Krebs, 2013; Dunbar, 2017; Dunbar & Barrett, 2007; Gilbert, 2019a; Nesse, 2019; Panksepp, 1998; Sapolsky, 2017; Zeigler-Hill, Welling, & Shackelford, 2015). Linking evolution dispositions with life history and maturation trajectories, which vary according to social contexts, gives insight into the sources of a range of mental health difficulties as well as prosocial and antisocial behaviours (Del Giudice, 2016). Indeed, we now know that social contexts can actually shape our genetic expressions, the genes that get turned on and off in us (Cowan, Callaghan, Kan, & Richardson, 2016).

## *Trade-offs, compromises and constraints*

What is crucial to the EFA is the recognition that evolution doesn't build organisms that are designed to be happy, 'mentally well' or always prosocial. Evolution can even create physical forms that don't function that well. This is because evolution is driven by building organisms that pursue survival and reproductive strategies, but in the process there are trade-offs where an advantage in one area can give disadvantages in another. The classic example of a problematic trade-off is the evolution of walking upright and hands-free, which had the downside of narrowing the female birth canal just at the time when the baby's head was evolving to get larger. The unfortunate consequence is that humans have the most dangerous and painful births of all primates. Consider another problematic trade-off, human cognitive competencies. These make it possible for us to be extraordinary in how we impact the world and pursue our survival and reproductive strategies. But they have made us into a species of extremes (Gilbert, 1989, 2018;

Marsh, 2019). We are the most caring of species, not only within close relationships but in professions like medicine. Yet for every pound we spend on medical research we spend far more on tribal violence. We are a terrifying, sadistic and destructive species with our inventions of horrendous ways of killing and torturing each other, the Roman games, the Holocaust and slavery to mention some of the most obvious. These are all consequences of trade-offs arising from the advantages and disadvantages of human intelligence linking up with evolutionary old motivational processes (Gilbert, 2018; Sapolsky, 2017).

Importantly, adaptive function can easily become dysregulated and dysfunctional. For example, diarrhoea and vomiting are the body's natural way of removing toxins; they are adapted defences and are not the 'illness' (Nesse, 2019). However, when they become dysregulated people will die from dehydration and nutrient loss. The down-regulation of positive emotion as occurs in depression and various anxieties can be seen as useful defences in some contexts. But they can become dysfunctional, particularly in a mind that is able to consciously experience its own mental states, consider its future and ruminate on stressful themes (Gilbert, 1992).

Another aspect of evolution is that it doesn't always go well, because it has to work with major constraints from what's gone before. It cannot go back to the drawing board and start again even if the basic design is no longer that adaptive. Evolution can't suddenly design a completely different skeleton which would be better for upright walking and wouldn't give us the associated hip, knee or human birthing difficulties. Given the high prevalence and incidence of mental health problems, not to mention forms of antisocial and immoral behaviour, evolutionary approaches address the issue explored by many evolutionary theorists, and was the subject of a paper over 20 years ago of 'Why isn't the mind better designed than it is?' (Gilbert, 1998). Strategies that are primarily intended for gene survival and reproduction/replication, along with organisms that are built with trade-offs, compromises and constraints, are part of the answer.

Serious too is the way that modern environments, of megacities with multiple strangers that we have created because of our intelligence, are now contexts that can bring out the worst in us; increasing social wariness and intensifying self-focused competitive psychology and tribal violence (Gilbert, 2018; Sapolsky, 2017). So EFA has little trouble with social constructivist approaches to motivation and emotion that highlight their contextual processes, flexibility and variation (Barrett, 2017; Zeigler-Hill et al., 2015). Many phenotypes for psychosocial functioning are highly sensitive to social contexts in regard to their expression (Sapolsky, 2017). This makes social contextualism powerful because it choreographs our needs, motives and algorithms that are wired into our brains.

EFA also suggests that concepts like depression are abstract concepts, with dubious reliability in terms of specific syndromes. What is important are the highly variable underlying processes that give rise to those mental states we label depression. Indeed, Akiskal and McKinney (1973) wrote a very influential paper on the heterogeneity of depression highlighting the fact that depressed states represented *final common pathways* from multiple interacting factors.

EFA can help distinguish between genuine pathologies (e.g., dementias; deficient B12) and variations in phenotypic function in response to environmental contingencies, particularly along dimensions of prosperities verses adversities (Nesse, 2019; Nesse & Williams, 1995). This is reminiscent of Hill's (1968) famous question of whether depression is a 'reaction posture or disease' which is still debated today (Gilbert, 2006). Given that most concepts of depression place loss of positive affect central to the difficulty, and indeed my PhD studies supported that, then the evolutionary question would be: what is the adaptive value of toning down positive affect and reward sensitivity, reducing explorative behaviour and confidence, suppressing aggression and becoming behaviourally wary and inhibited? Are there particular contexts where this pattern of responding is likely? And looking at other associated experiences: what is the adaptive value of seeing oneself as inferior or disconnected from others? Asking these questions doesn't mean we are arguing that psychiatric syndromes or psychiatric labels are adaptive. EFA does not ask what the adaptive function of 'depression' is because that's a complex, variant and heterogeneous syndrome. Rather it considers the potential adaptive value of subcomponents, in what contexts might they be adaptive and in what contexts may they become maladaptive to turn down spirit of behaviour and positive reward sensitivity. Before thinking of depression as a pathology we need to think about how some of its elements represent defensive strategies subject to genetic, epigenetic and contextual variation. Such mental states, with these subcomponents, should be noted in other species, and the contexts in which they are generated should have some degree of cross species consistency. That then is the background for the research to be discussed.

## *EFA candidates for depression*

There have been many candidates suggested as the core candidates for evolved mechanisms underpinning depression (reviewed elsewhere Gilbert, 1992, 2006, 2007, 2013). One of the earliest ideas was that the depressed-like states are ways of conserving resources in poor payoff environments; that is when invigorated efforts are likely to fail then it's better to reduce activity. One hunkers down and waits for better times. Nesse (2000) offered an updated model of this approach. Linked, but also different, were studies looking at what happens to animals who are confronted by stresses they could not control. This evolved into the *learned helplessness model* of depression suggesting when stress first occurs there is an invigorated effort to try to escape or control it. If, and when, those efforts and struggles fail, and the animal learns that nothing they do will work, explorative and effortful behaviour is switched off, they close down outputs and become withdrawn, passive and inhibited (Peterson, Maier, & Seligman, 1993; Seligman, 1975). These are not consciously chosen strategies but ways in which the physiological system reacts to that kind of stress. Debate arose as to whether this was a learnt phenomenon, or a biological phenomenon related to (for example) monoamine depletion associated with fear, stress and other factors (Weiss, Demetrikopoulos, McCurdy, West, & Bonsall, 2000). Indeed, much earlier, Hans Selye (1936) had proposed a model for stress called General Adaptation Syndrome. Here, the first response is recognition of the threat that alarms and activates the sympathetic stress flight and fight system. If this continues the body tries to resist by parasympathetic regulation and bringing the state back into balance but when this fails, the body enters a state of exhaustion and depletion. So, exhaustion can be produced by both the failed coping efforts of the organism and the degree of extended stress. Hence, running away from a lion is over pretty quickly whereas being trapped in an abusive marriage is an extensive, prolonged stressor. Although females of various species have to cope with aggressive males from time to time there is nothing in nature like being trapped in abusive or hostile marriages for months and sometimes years on end; there is nothing in nature that traps us in jobs we hate or fear losing. In fact, we have created *a world of traps* for many aspects of our everyday life where we are finding ourselves having to do things when we don't really want to and find stressful over the longer term (Gilbert, 2018; Ryan, 2019). These are completely abnormal contexts. The paradox is that we can create contexts with an evolved mind that we weren't actually evolved to function within! Importantly, what all these models share is that threats and stressors trigger a triphasic response pattern where the first defence is to increase energy expenditure, effort and struggle, but 'if nothing is working' (then there is a switch to closing outputs down and) 'do nothing" (Gilbert, 1984, 1988). A third phase may well be adaptation or gradual recovery. The cognitive therapies also highlight how cognitions could interact with this process. This is partly because our capacity for having objective self-awareness and ability to think about the future means that we can ruminate on themes that constantly stimulate threat and stress processing systems. These forms of rumination prevent the body from moving into a rest and digest recovering and resetting system (Gilbert, 2019a).

What was also important for this model was that these learned helplessness states could be conditioned. For example pairing a particular light with uncontrollable stress produced helplessness states that could reactivate helpless states when presented (see Gilbert, 1992 for a review). These classical conditioning learning models are profoundly important for understanding how 'the body remembers' and can be quickly activated into different patterns through associative learning.

## The social dynamics of depression

### *Attachment*

Important though these stress-control models are, they didn't address some of the social behaviours and cognitions associated with depression (Gilbert, 1992, 2006, 2007). These included a sense of isolation and loneliness on the one hand, and tendencies towards inferiority (unfavourable social comparison), submissive behaviour, poor assertiveness and shame and self-criticism on the other. There was no clear reason why people experiencing uncontrollable stresses would end up feeling worthless, inferior and shame prone. We needed a theory that illuminated the social dynamics, social motives and social cognitions of depression. Maybe the type of stress that was producing inhibited-helpless states was important and would texture the defensive response?

Two social theories of depression that implicitly incorporated learned helplessness type concepts, but focused on different types of *social* threat and stressor, were the attachment and loss model (Bowlby, 1969, 1973,

1980; see Cassidy & Shaver, 2016; Music, 2019 for reviews) and the social competition (Price, 1972; Price, Sloman, Gardner, Gilbert, & Rohde, 1994) and defeat and entrapment models (Dixon, 1998; Dixon, Fisch, Huber, & Walser, 1989; Gilbert, 1984, 1992, 2007; Gilbert & Allan, 1998). The attachment and loss model posits that mammals, and especially humans, are motivated to form attachments with caring others in early life and then throughout life seek to elicit support, guidance and help from others. These relationships have powerful physiological regulating effects. When these are forthcoming individuals feel safe and confident, are able to explore and develop, whereas when these are not available, and individuals feel in unsupportive, neglectful, critical/hostile social environments they are vulnerable to unregulated stress and mental health problems. Humans have basic needs for support and connectedness. The presence of supportive others suppresses threat and stress processing (see Cassidy & Shaver, 2016; Music, 2019 for reviews). For example, partner support is associated with reduced cortisol and increased oxytocin when facing stress Grewen, Girdler, Amico, & Light, 2005; Heinrichs, Baumgartner, Kirschbaum, & Ehlert, 2003; for a review see Petrocchi & Cheli, 2019).

In early life a range of complex needs for food, comfort protection and stimulation is provided to the infant by the mother. So crucial is this relationship that they have evolved monitoring systems to keep tabs on each other's closeness and availability. Given the survival imperative to elicit care from the parent a set of monitoring and defensive manoeuvres for when these are disrupted evolved. These relate to a menu of potentially achieving mechanisms and defensive/protective motivational, emotional and behavioural control systems that serve the function of keeping an infant and mother in close contact with each other (Bowlby, 1969). When separated from their mother, juveniles lose these vital maternal inputs and are at risk from a variety of dangers to which they must now be attentive and respond. The defensive response to separation is *protest-despair*. Protest is (as in the learned helplessness model) an invigorated pattern of responding with specific social attention to engage in urgent searching for the parent and to *signal/communicate* distress to elicit help and/or reunion; i.e., the signal is designed to impact on others. But if this doesn't work, in the sense that it doesn't elicit reunion or caring behaviour from the (m)other, then this 'noisy' defensive behaviour actually becomes a threat because it increases the risk of signalling its defencelessness to predators, getting lost and getting dehydrated. So, after a period there is an internal process to shut the infant down and generate hiding behaviour and wait for parental rescue. Despair is a form of behavioural deactivation when protest does not work, and similar to the inhibited states noted in learned helplessness. Despair is thus designed to *stop signalling* and moving in the environment (hunker down) when not to do so is dangerous (for reviews see Cassidy & Shaver, 2016).

Although these are the basic templates and algorithms of defences, they become extraordinarily complex in contexts of disrupted attachment. This is where children are subject to frequent separations, abandonment, neglect or abuse. In the latter case the parent, who should be the source of a secure base and safe haven, is a source of threat, creating serious approach-avoidance conflicts for the infant. This results in the child experiencing 'threat without resolution' because the threatening parent also robs the child of their means of confident resolution via contact with a caring other (Liotti, 2000). This can underpin disorganised attachment (Blizard, 2003). There is not space here to engage in detailed discussions of the maturation of attachment mechanisms and defences under different conditions, but they are profoundly important, not least because individuals can experience rapid switching between protest/activation and despair/deactivation states as part of their mental health problem. These insights have also underpinned explorations of the mechanisms by which compassion focused therapy can reactivate attachment process so they can function as a secure base and safe haven (Gilbert, 2000).

## *Hierarchy, social power and rank*

Importantly, the need to hunker down and give up on exploration and resource seeking could also be triggered in another social context. This is one linked to problems with social competition, status and low rank. Again evolution seems to have given a set of defences for coping with this scenario. This is the social competition hypothesis of depression that had not received much research attention at the time (Price, 1972; Price & Sloman, 1987; Price et al., 1994). This approach noted that in contexts of competing for social and other resources, constant fighting with risk of injury is costly, particularly in small groups where there may be genetic relationships. Hence, two strategies evolved. One is to escalate conflict until winning; the other, in the face of likely injury or defeat, is to de-escalate, submit, withdraw and signal to the more powerful that one is no longer a threat. Technically this was called the *involuntary subordinate strategy* (Sloman & Gilbert, 2000). To run this strategy a whole range of physiological systems has to be demobilised so that reward and exploratory-seeking systems are toned down or deactivated, while submissive inhibition is turned on. Again we can see the basic learned helplessness blueprint here but that triggers are specific to social conflict. If a dominant sees a subordinate seeking resources including sexual opportunities (their drive system is active) they will threaten and even attack the subordinate. Evolution thus evolved mechanisms that enabled individuals, who are at risk of hostilities from more powerful others, to monitor themselves in relation to others closely and to express submissive and defeat-like behaviours (Gilbert, 2000; Price, 2000). Such behaviours, in contrast to (say) defiant displays, can terminate the attack impulses in the more powerful. Threatened subordinates need to remain anxiously vigilant to dominant others, and reduce confident and explorative behaviours. Some studies suggest that if they don't, for example, if juveniles become overly challenging, they can be attacked by more dominant individuals and killed (Higley et al., 1996). These important components of social defensive behaviours could play a role in depression vulnerability and presentation because they directly link to social wariness, loss of confidence and reduced reward seeking and explorative behaviour.

John Price and Leon Sloman, who became friends and mentors, and I became very interested in exploring if it was indeed competitive motivational systems that utilised evolved mechanisms for monitoring and judging social rank and social threat that were being triggered in depression (Gilbert, 1984, 1992). Particularly important might be the mechanisms track for signals of social comparison, potential for social conflict, rejection and unwanted low rank. The basic idea was that problems in navigating one's social place and position can manifest as being in unwanted inferior positions, with low social control over access to positive resources, reduced support and investment from others. In addition people can feel trapped in these aversive, rejecting critical situations and relationships. These contextual cues would then (unintentionally) trigger subordinate defences.

Just as attachment, connectedness and access to support and help from others is a fundamental human motive system so is the need for status (see Anderson, Hildreth, & Howland, 2015). As such it has its own algorithms and orientations. Part of the motive and advantages of status is that it opens access to these valuable resources, social esteem, opportunities to have supportive friends and good reproductive partners, which as noted have physiological regulating effects. People will try and avoid low status if the consequence of low status is loss of these. If (in certain contexts and roles) low status doesn't carry such costs then it's less likely to be intensified as a motive. Anderson, Kraus, Galinsky, and Keltner (2012) showed that it is *social* status, relating to how one is held in the minds of others, one's social reputation, degree of attractiveness and interest to others, rather than socio economic status, that is linked to well-being. Self-esteem relates to having qualities that you feel *others will value* rather than devalue or be indifferent to. It became clear then that one couldn't consider competitive theories of depression without considering *what* is being competed for. That question highlights the interconnectedness between social competition and the drive for social connectedness and social influence.

## *Competing for what?*

While humans can of course compete aggressively as in bullying and domestic violence which are linked to depression, many researchers point out that most forms of human competition are about reputation, being attractive to others and social standing (Barkow, 1975; Sznycer et al., 2018). I labelled this *social attention holding potential* (SAHP) (Gilbert, 1989, 1992, 1997; Gilbert, Price, & Allan, 1995). Indeed, given we have a basic motivation for 'status', (Anderson et al., 2015) for which monitoring the SAHP is central, Boksem, Kostermans, Milivojevic, and De Cremer (2011) showed that we have status-attention monitoring systems. Low status individuals monitor status in a different way from high status individuals. One of the reasons for this is that low status individuals are much more vulnerable to downrank threats and losses, and have to be more vigilant (Gilbert, 1995). Evolution did not develop new defences according to the type of competition any more than there is a different anxiety system for an approaching lion, losing one's passport at an airport or hearing of the serious illness of your partner. They will all operate through the amygdala in some way, although the coping behaviours will be quite different, of course. So monitoring SAHP, status and reputation are linked into much earlier evolved defences of activation and deactivation according to the success or failure of competitive and status acquiring and maintaining efforts and contexts. Hence, social putdowns, rejections and being marginalised/ignored are forms of social diminishment that could trigger subordinate defences of involuntary subordinate strategies (Sloman, 2000). The concept of SAHP, linked to attention monitoring, offered a bridge into the attachment-loss dimensions of depression, in that failure to compete for social place resulted in rejection and loss of access to the positive regulating effects of supportive and caring relationships. It also bridges into the shame literature in that at the heart of shame is a sense of social diminishment as a result of losing SAHP or having negative SAHP and being an object of derision and negative evaluation by others (Gilbert, 2007).

A second question about competing and striving was the degree to which these were to get 'well above others', seek superiority or whether they were competing to avoid inferiority and rejection. Social disconnection, and being cut off from helpful others, is a major evolutionary threat. In the past being shunned, excluded, rejected and abandoned individuals wouldn't survive. So the research set out on a series of studies exploring striving and competing *to avoid inferiority*, and associated fear of losing out and being rejected for failure (Gilbert et al., 2007, 2009; Basran, Pires, Matos, McEwan, & Gilbert, 2019). This was running true to our basic approach to always explore functions behind these processes. The data turned out to be as predicted. Depression and anxiety were linked to striving, competitiveness to avoid inferiority and its consequences such as rejection and marginalisation. The *functions* of achievement, striving and competitiveness are crucial. It is when they are driven via social insecurity, efforts to prove oneself to others and avoid loss of social investment from one's local relationships, that vulnerability to mental health problems arise. In some sense then striving and competitiveness, with its focus on social comparison, are strategic efforts to avoid the survival threat of loss of social interest and investment from others, or outright rejection. This approach has considerable overlaps with studies of perfectionism and the link of perfectionistic processes to excessive competitiveness and competitive-status anxiety which has been growing in the last 20 years (Curran & Hill, 2019). Here was another bridge linking striving and competitiveness to issues of attachment, social (inter)connectedness and social support. What's different for humans is that other primates are not desperately trying to prove their attractiveness, talents or value to others. This is very much a human competitive domain emerging from the need for social connectedness, being desired and acceptance and the physiological, psychological and practical benefits that flow from that (Gilbert, 2007, 2019b).

There is increasing evidence that neoliberalism is a factor that has unhelpfully accentuated competitive motivation particularly in younger cohorts who are caught up in increasing levels of anxiety and depression (Curran & Hill, 2019). As these researchers highlight the fear of being marginalised if one can't keep up or present oneself in a certain way has soaked through our culture. Narcissistic anxieties have increased too, while concern for others has lessened (Curran & Hill, 2019)

## *Shame*

Competing for social status, sense of belonging and social investment from others opens up the concern with its opposite, shame. I wrote an early piece on distinguishing shame from guilt on the basis of different evolutionary mechanisms (Gilbert, 1988). Shame is linked to status competition whereas guilt (the feeling of sadness and remorse for causing harm) evolved as a harm avoidance and reparation motivation with the evolution of caring (for reviews see Gilbert, 2019b). Shame can also be distinguished in terms of being externally and internally focused (Gilbert, 1998, 2019b). External shame is focused on the experience of negative evaluation from others whereas internal shame is linked to self-criticism and self-devaluation (Gilbert, 2007). This distinction is now utilised in a number of different models of shame. In a meta-analysis Kim, Thibodeau, and Jorgensen (2011) confirmed this as an important distinction and found that external shame was a good predictor of depression and anxiety.

## *Defeats*

However, the focus on (only) subordinate defences also fitted with social anxiety and other mental health difficulties (Gilbert, 2000, 2001). The social competition theory, and later what I referred to as *social rank theory* (partly because it was perceptions of social rank that ecological research focused on and we developed our self-report measures for) (Gilbert, 1992), suggested that *in*voluntary subordinate states may well be vulnerability factors for depression. But what triggered them? This was not dissimilar to Brown and Harris' (1978) idea that we can distinguish between vulnerability factors and provoking agents/triggers. So what was needed to trigger a depressed state was either chronic stress and/or some kind of (social) defeat (Price, 1972; Price & Sloman, 1987). Fearful subordinates might well be stressed, but they aren't necessarily depressed. However, if they experience down rank attacks they cannot defend against, are hustled, bullied, harassed and defeated they would be vulnerable to depressed states ( Dixon et al., 1989; Dixon, 1998; Gilbert, 1992, 2001).

Defeats can make people vulnerable to depression for a number of reasons. First, defeats could be like learned helplessness. Individuals struggled against adversity, but when they could not avoid, escape or control it, the next best defence was to hunker down and stop struggling. A second idea was linked to disengagement from pointless or hopeless tasks, or tasks that could result in serious injury if the individual continued. Another idea was if a defeat required major adaptation over the long term, people's perception of an aversive or loss filled future might trigger a low energy expenditure strategy. Another idea was that the display of defeat states, with loss of muscle tone and body posture, was a signal to an aggressor that one is now weak, out of action and not a threat. The classic display would be the defeated army; indeed, defeats over important conflicts regularly produce diminishment of mood and energy. Finally, given that social defeats can also be about social disengagement (feeling worthless and socially disengaged and lonely) then they may also trigger protest-despair type defences. Indeed, many clients have noted that they often have 'inner ideals' they are trying to live up to, thinking that reaching these ideas will make them socially accepted and reduce risk of marginalisation. If they persistently fail to reach their ideals there can be an overwhelming sense of being defeated and engaged in struggles one can't win. However such defeats go with a sense of failure and feeling inferior associated with a sense of disconnection and loneliness and being cut off or excluded from the core valuable social inputs that regulate threat processing; that is when mental health problems emerge. Again it can be stressed that defeats that don't have these consequences are less likely to be pathogenic (Sturman, Rose, McKeighan, Burch, & Evanico, 2015).

## *Entrapments*

Another major difference between us and other primates is that humans are far more 'caged' (in houses and families) and are not free roaming like most primates who can distance themselves from aggressive others (Ryan, 2019). Thus, as we can't get away from contexts where we have experienced defeat, the concept of entrapment became important too.

When individuals are trapped and want to get away from situations, they become 'flight orientated'. But if they are in some way trapped and can't execute the flight strategy and behavioural routine then they are in a state of arrested defences, called 'arrested flight' ( Dixon et al., 1989; Dixon, 1998). Over time arrested flight could produce inhibited and demobilised states, and in that sense is similar to learned helplessness (Gilbert, 1992, 2001). In addition, humans typically engage in what is called experiential avoidance where they try to get away from aversive memories, thoughts and feelings. We therefore extended this idea of 'entrapment with arrested flight' – an elevated motivation to escape, take flight from, and get rid of internal experiences. We called it internal entrapment. While this pertained to issues of rumination and feeling stuck and trapped in inner thoughts, feelings and mood states, the crucial issue was the degree to which individuals were flight motivated, trying to get away from, suppress or avoid having these experiences. Individuals are trying to get away from their own distressing mental states, thoughts and ruminations, but feel stuck and trapped in them. Brown and Harris (1978) published extensive research showing that the social contexts of women's lives significantly contributed to risk of depression. Following up on the social rank and entrapment model, they investigated and found that humiliation events (involving the loss of status and social power) and feeling trapped in aversive environments were major contributors to depression in women (Brown, Harris, & Hepworth, 1995).

So crucial too was the idea that even defeats might not result in depression if animals could:

1 *Escape the context, including the physical context.* When individuals can get away from bullying relations or abusive marriages/partnerships their depression tends to reduce and confidence improves.
2 *Be able to give up on a pursuit and do something else.* When individuals experience major losses and defeats in life, their ability to find new meaning and rewarding activities can be crucial to recovery. If they stay stuck in grieving and feeling defeated for what's been lost, depression can become more stuck. This can be a problem where individuals feel they weren't properly parented and constantly seek to find a parenting caring relationship.
3 *Be able to elicit support and caring.* In primates access to supportive (and grooming) others offsets the impact of social threat, defeat or attack (Abbott et al., 2004). Similarly eliciting social support and care in the face of defeats and setbacks can offset their impact on depressed states (Brugha, 1995).

### *Self-monitoring and social mentalities*

Biological systems have a built-in monitoring process that will trigger particular reactions in certain contexts. For example, if the temperature goes too high we start to sweat. If it goes too low we start to shiver. If we take in toxins the stomach detects this and then triggers expulsions as vomiting. We don't learn these; they are biologically built-in, basic algorithms. Just as we have these basic *biological* monitoring systems we have ones for monitoring self in relationship to others in the social arenas of life. We have systems that can monitor how we are doing in relationship to others. This monitoring is partly focused on monitoring and evaluating the intent and motivation from others towards the self and how our communications of intent and motives are influencing the minds of others.

In order for animals to form any kind of reciprocal role, be it for sexual relations, cooperation, attachment and so forth individuals have to be able to monitor their own outputs in relationship to the behaviours of the other; to their conspecifics. Social behaviour requires coordinated interactions for these interpersonal dances. The attachment system the child has will monitor the availability and accessibility of the parent. Crudely, the monitoring system is 'parent present and available then suppress threat system'; 'parent not present or available activate threat arousal and seeking behaviour'. Physiologically the presence of the parent stimulates the vagal brake and the absence of the parent releases that brake (Porges, 2017). A distal but nevertheless related experience is that when we feel lonely we want to contact somebody we like or think cares about us; loneliness is the feeling that will trigger desires/motives to seek connectedness. So our self-to-other monitoring system is biologically plugged in to our emotions for threat awareness, drive and reward, and safeness (Gilbert, 2019a). How we monitor our sense of social acceptability and connectedness is very much tuned by our early life experiences, but the point is that we are monitoring how we are existing in the mind of others.

If individuals are indeed being triggered into involuntary subordinate strategies, then the internal monitoring system will not be telling them how confident they are, how strong they are and how likely they are to succeed if they just keep going; quite the opposite. A threatened subordinate in the wild who was not controlled by this evaluative and warning system would get hammered! The monitoring system will be giving thoughts and feelings that incline them to back off, that they are weaker, they can't achieve the outcome and risk getting injured. If you then textured this with actual (early life) experiences of being criticised and bullied then you have a very powerful internal regulator because they are tuned to subordinate strategies and will be playing memories of putdown, loss and attack.

## Self-criticism

This raises an important theme relating to self-criticism. In social conflict situations, when an animal realises they are in an inferior position and have to submit to avoid injury, there has to be some monitoring system that tells them they are the weaker member. John Price called this *the internal referee* of social competition. It operates physiologically to turn off engagement systems and turn on submissive subordinate systems (the involuntary subordinate strategy). Having a monitoring system that basically is conveying information 'you can do this. . . , but you can't do that. . .'; 'if you try to do this (make a sexual advance) then you will be attacked by powerful others' could well be an early blueprint for self-criticism. Clearly self-criticism is considerably more complex but it operates like some judge of competence and ability. Clients quickly pick up that self-criticism is much more intense in contexts of status threat and concerns inferiority and rejection. In a series of studies Fournier, Moskowitz and Zuroff (2002) showed that in organisational settings individuals who felt inferior tended to be quarrelsome with those below them but submitted more and inhibited anger more to those above.

Another aspect of these basic defences is the way in which they have become linked into self-monitoring systems. It is well known that we can create images in our minds that stimulate the same physiological pathways as the unconditioned stimulus. For example, feeling hungry and seeing a wonderful meal or just *imagining* a wonderful meal stimulates the same hypothalamic pathways. Seeing something sexual or imagining something sexual stimulates the same physiological pathways. It is therefore possible for us to create internal images of ourselves and the world where we feel inferior and trapped and thus stimulate those defences. Given that the social rank and defeat defences were designed to deal with hostile signals from others, then if we generate those in ourselves in the form of self-criticism it's quite possible that our own hostile self-criticism can stimulate the defensive pathways (Gilbert, 1992, 2000). Indeed we have good neurophysiological evidence for this now (Longe et al., 2010). To put it simply self-criticism operates through the same physiological systems, activating the same strategies as criticism/threat from a dominant other. Once owned self-criticism can stimulate involuntary subordinate strategies and over time a relentless sense of defeat and loneliness. These two constantly run together because individuals who feel defeated but well-loved and connected are less vulnerable to depression.

There is considerable work on self-criticism and its link to a range of pathologies (Kannan & Levitt, 2013). In addition, some years ago I noted that even when people are trying to generate positive and helpful statements for the self as in cognitive therapy, the emotional tones and texture of those thoughts could still be hostile. Indeed, the basis of compassion focused therapy began by trying to help people generate supportive, kind and compassionate emotional *motives, tones and textures* in their own coping thoughts rather than hostile ones (Gilbert, 1998, 2000, 2019a). So in effect it wasn't (just) the cognitive content but the emotional tone of people's self-monitoring thoughts that was impacting physiological systems. What EFA allows is the potential to see how and why the signals we create in our minds, and the internal models of self and the world we create, stimulate these basic physiological patterns of various social defences.

Exploring the interaction between these processes, Sturman and Mongrain (2005) found that self-reported entrapment and unfavourable social comparison mediated effect of self-criticism on the number of previous episodes of depression. Feeling inferior compared to others, self-criticalness and feeling trapped in that position are particularly depressogenic.

## Summary

This research tradition has followed an EFA approach exploring how two fundamental survival and reproductive motivational systems operate as physiological and psychological regulators. The first is linked to how individuals compete for resources and create different types of hierarchies which are linked to different types of monitoring and self-evaluative systems and physiologies. For example, social rank systems utilise forms of social comparison, sensitivity to self-other competencies and menus for enacting dominant-submissive behaviour. Mammals also need the help of others to survive and therefore have a range of evolved physiological and psychological processes that are regulated

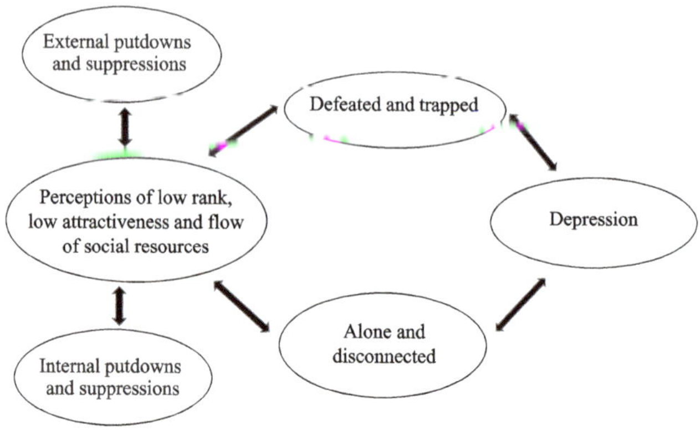


**FIGURE 1.1** Simple interaction between rank and social connectedness for depression (copyright P. Gilbert)

via the helpfulness or otherwise of relationships. Research over the last 30 years has shown how these systems interact and become major regulators of a range of process underpinning mental health problems. One of the crucial implications of this approach is how sensitive our minds and bodies are to their embedded social contexts (Gilbert, 1995). After all, evolution has been all about developing mechanisms of being sensitive to social context and the co-creation of social roles.

Figure 1.1 gives a simple overview of these processes.

It starts with the idea that external putdowns, criticisms, rejections and being bullied through to forms of abuse, sensitise individuals monitoring of the social rank and relative power; their abilities to be connected and valued social agents. In addition, individuals can experience considerable suppression of desired goals because of operating in demanding or toxic environments. For example, individuals who desperately want to get away from stressful jobs or marriages but can't afford to. These are forms of arrested defences which have overlaps with the learned helplessness literature (Gilbert, 2001). Part of this suppression is also the inability to form or unavailability to form helpful connectedness with others.

Individuals can also experience considerable internal putdowns, for example, from replaying trauma memories, or hostile self-criticism. Social and paranoid anxieties may suppress people's social reward seeking and relationship developing behaviours. These drive a sense of being defeated and trapped and at the same time an awareness of lacking social resources and sense of disconnectedness. Given that social resources in the forms of socially connectedness, sense of belonging and feeling cared about and cared for, have powerful physiological effects to dampen the threat system, being cut off from them has health implications. In effect having a sense of connectedness and a valued sense of status and control, increases the sense of 'being in safe environments' which operate through systems like the vagal nerve (Petrocchi & Cheli, 2019) and can suppress threat processing (Kelly, Zuroff, Leybman, & Gilbert, 2012).

## Underpinning research and scales development

Evolutionary psychology is now a flourishing, rich and multivariate discipline (Buss, 2015; Dunbar, 2017; Dunbar & Barrett, 2007; Zeigler-Hill et al., 2015). Over the last 40 years there's also been a gradual movement to use EFA to investigate the different motivational systems that orientate individuals to life strategies making them vulnerable to mental health problems, antisocial behaviour or increase prosocial behaviour (Brüne, 2015; Chua, Lukaszewski, Grant, & Sng, 2016; Gilbert, 1989, 1998, 2019a; McGuire & Troisi, 1998; Nesse, 2019).

### *Social rank measures*

What was lacking however were self-report scales that could tap into the dynamics of social competition linked to low rank states (Gilbert, 1984, 1989, 1992). So Steve Allan and I started to develop a set of self-report scales that could tap three core aspects of perceived social rank. These were: 1. a social comparison scale based on a Likert measure (Allan & Gilbert, 1995); 2. a submissive behaviours scale derived from the work of Buss and Craik (1986) and 3. an external shame scale exploring the degree to which people thought others saw them as inferior, flawed or inadequate (Allan, Gilbert, & Goss, 1994; Goss, Gilbert, & Allan, 1994). We distinguished submissive behaviour from assertiveness and found that depression was highly correlated with self-reported submissive behaviour and lower assertiveness (Allan & Gilbert, 1997; Gilbert & Allan, 1994).

### *Shame measures*

Although some shame researchers focused on self-evaluation and exposure others are more social and contextual, arguing that we experience shame from how we feel *others* perceive and react to us. This is in line with sociologist Cooley's (1902) concept of *the looking glass self* whereby we experience ourselves positively or negatively according to how we sense we exist in the minds of others. The child does not experience shame until they are made aware of some negative social judgement about some attribute of self, as judged in the mind of another. Being judged negatively (looked down on or seen as inferior, rejectable or worthy of attack) is obviously a dimension of social rank theory. Therefore, we set about developing measures for external shame (the other as shamer scale; OAS) and sought to distinguish it from internal shame (Gilbert, 1992; Goss et al., 1994; Allan et al., 1994). The scale has now been used in many studies. Kim et al. (2011) published a major meta-analysis and review that demonstrated that external shame was indeed a powerful predictor of depression and other forms of psychopathology.

## *Types of inferiority*

When it comes to feeling inferior and low rank we were interested in whether this was experienced for all qualities of self, as might be implied by the generalised global self-esteem literature, or only in those domains where one felt unable *to compete* for resources and social place. For example, do depressed people see themselves as inferior when it comes to prosocial traits such as being caring, trustworthy or helpful? The answer seems to be 'no they don't' especially when controlling for submissiveness. It is in the resource control and dynamics of life that depressed people see themselves as inferior (McEwan, Gilbert, & Duarte, 2012).

## *Measuring defeat and entrapment*

As noted, the issue of defeat and entrapment had always been prominent and explicit within the social rank model. Hence, in 1998 we developed the social defeat and entrapment questionnaires to explore people's sense of being defeated by life and in relationships (Gilbert & Allan, 1998). Our 1998 paper showed that in both student and depressed populations external and internal entrapment are highly associated with depression. In the depressed group they are also highly correlated with hopelessness. Interestingly, internal entrapment (feeling trapped in states of mind and thinking that one wanted to escape from) had a slightly higher correlation (r = .62) to depression than external (r = .54). To some extent this also overlaps with concepts such as experiential avoidance, a wanting to get away from one's feelings, memories and intrusive thoughts. The association of depression with defeat was .73 in the students and .77 in the depressed population. In a follow-up study, Gilbert, Allan, Brough, Melly, and Miles (2002) explored self-report measures of social rank variables including social comparison, submissive behaviour and external shame along with defeat and entrapment in relationship to anhedonia and anxiety in 81 inpatients and 193 undergraduates. Depression was highly correlated with rank variables and once again in the clinical group anhedonia and anxiety were strongly correlated with entrapment (r = .63) and defeat (r = .79).

The study of defeat and entrapment states has now been replicated all over the world using our scales and various hybrids (Taylor, Gooding, Wood, & Tarrier, 2011; Sturman et al., 2015). Unlike Taylor, Wood, Gooding, Johnson, and Tarrier (2009), who argued for a single factor combining defeat and entrapment, Höller et al. (2020) developed a short version of a scale combining defeat and entrapment scale and tested it on a large group of out and inpatients. They found two clear separate factors. Suicidal ideators and suicide attempters scored significantly higher on entrapment in defeat than non/low ideators and attempters.

In 2004, Gilbert, Gilbert and Irons explored life events using the *life events and difficulties schedule* of Brown and Harris (1978) in 50 depressed patients. In regard to arrested flight, 88% of the group acknowledged strong desires to escape difficulties in their life but most felt unable to. Transcript analysis from the LEDS also indicated strong themes of entrapment. It found 38.7% felt trapped before becoming depressed. Feeling trapped by the depression itself (no energy to do anything) was also an issue. Fantasies of escaping were common, but making actual plans to get away less common, possibly because that was anxiety provoking. A variety of reasons was given for not escaping. In regard to arrested anger, 82% felt they suppressed their anger and 56% felt this problem predated their depression.

Recently these concepts have been used to develop a semi-structured interview for people who have suicidal ideation and have engaged in self harm. The study was conducted in an accident and emergency service for people who had recently self-harmed. Both clinicians and clients found that a sense of entrapment, arrested flight and arrested fight were very prominent in these individuals. Interestingly, thinking about and discussing these themes with clinicians was viewed as very helpful (Clarke et al., 2016).

### *Competing to avoid inferiority*

As noted earlier understanding how and what people are competing for, and the fears of failure to be able to compete, was the driving force behind the fears and inferiority studies. Again, we pioneered some of the scales for that measurement (Gilbert, Broomhead et al., 2007; Gilbert, McEwan et al., 2009).

## The transition from pure research to application

There have been many studies using these scales and confirming that submissive behaviour, feeling inferior in the eyes of others and unfavourable social comparisons are highly linked to depression, social anxiety and other mental health problems. Wetherall, Robb, and O'Connor (2019) conducted a major systematic review of the data for social rank theory finding good evidence from many sources showing these are salient issues of depression. What is central for mental health problems is *in*voluntary and unwanted subordination. If we are happy being in lower ranking positions, which sometimes we are of course, especially if we feel others above us are helpful and supportive, then depression doesn't follow. It's only when the rank is associated with aversive outcomes that problems arise. This is because it triggers social defensive mechanisms in a way that being happy in a subordinate position obviously does not.

Taylor et al. (2011) provided a systematic review on a large body of evidence investigating the links among defeat, entrapment and psychopathology in the domains of depression, suicidality and posttraumatic stress disorder (PTSD). In the case of PTSD they looked at the concept of mental defeat and its prediction of severity and recovery. More recently Carvalho et al. (2013) further explored the relationship between entrapment, defeat and depression in nonclinical and depressed patients again supporting the strong association between entrapment and defeat in depression. Sturman and his colleges have also generated a number of studies developing the social rank theory of mood disorders. In a recent study Sturman et al. (2015; which also offers a review of their pioneering work) found that self-criticism was linked to increased sensitivity to defeat and number of perceived defeating events. Griffiths, Wood, Maltby, Taylor, and Tai (2014) showed that defeat and entrapment were highly predictive of depression and anxiety 12 months later. Griffiths, Wood, and Tai (2018) found that defeat and entrapment are predictors of depression and burden in carers; defeat and entrapment have also been shown to be important in other mental health difficulties such as psychosis (Valmaggia et al., 2015). Selten, van der Ven, Rutten, and Cantor-Graae (2013) gave an update on the social defeat model of psychosis including its overlap with animal models and neurophysiological pathways. Arrested defences and entrapped defeat states have also been linked to self-harm (Clarke et al., 2016). Siddaway, Taylor, Wood, and Schulz (2015) conducted a meta-analysis with over 40 studies (n = 10,072):

> Perceptions of defeat and entrapment were strong (around r = .60) and similar in size across all four psychiatric disorders. Perceptions of defeat were particularly strong in depression (r = .73). There was no between-study heterogeneity; therefore moderator analyses were conducted in an exploratory fashion. There was no evidence of publication bias.

The high correlation of over .7 of defeat with depression is now shown in many studies. As these authors suggest, defeat and entrapment may well be trans-diagnostic and should be a focus for therapeutic intervention.

## *Self-monitoring and self-criticism*

As noted earlier we can generate internal signals that stimulate natural defences. For example, anticipating, imagining or remembering a threat may be enough to stimulate the physiological pathways of the threat system, even in the absence of an actual threat stimulus. So the question was: could self-criticism be looked at this way; that is, can we generate internal signals that stimulate our social rank defences, particularly anxiety and demobilisation depressed states? Again we could keep the basic blueprint of learned helplessness, in the sense that attacks could first invigorate us and then if we don't succeed we get defeated, demoralised and demobilised (Whelton & Greenberg, 2005). Now this idea of self-criticism had been around for centuries (see Gilbert, 1992, for reviews). Freud (1917) argued that individuals, particularly children, could become fearful of expressing anger towards those they depended on because of the risk of counter-attack, rejection and disengagement. His idea was that the anger got directed to the self. This was called 'anger turned inward'. Freud was very influenced by Nietzsche, who argued that 'no one blames themselves without a secret wish for vengeance' (Ellenberger, 1970). As noted earlier there is now clear evidence that self-criticism, self-blame is linked to the nature of the rate relationship. Insofar as psychotic voice hearers can experience dominant critical voices attacking them Birchwood, Meaden, Trower, Gilbert, and Plaistow (2000) found that subordination to voices was closely linked to subordination and marginalization in other social relationships. In a study of people with schizophrenia who heard malevolent voices, and with self-critical depressed people, Gilbert et al. (2001) found

> evidence that . . . malevolent voice hearers and self-critical depressed people experience their hostile, internally generated voices/thoughts as powerful, dominating and controlling (i.e. have typical characteristics of a hostile dominant). Moreover, these voices/thoughts activate evolved subordinate defences such as fight/flight and these are associated with depression in both depression and schizophrenia.
>
> *(p. 1117)*

With the cognitive revolution, which saw self-criticism as forms of negative (cognitive) self-judgements, it became somewhat divorced from any underlying defensive motivation (for reviews see Gilbert & Irons, 2005). There is increasing evidence that perceptions of social rank have an impact on self-criticism (Sturman et al., 2015). Gilbert and Miles (2000) developed a measure called sensitivity to social put down and showed that individuals who felt inferior as measured by social comparison tended to blame themselves if they were criticised by others as those who had higher social comparison scores blamed others for being critical. Self-blame for being criticised by others was linked to psychopathologies variables.

In our research we wanted to explore both the forms *and* functions of self-criticism: not only why people self-criticise but also how. So we developed a self-criticism scale to do this (Gilbert, Clarke, Kempel, Miles, & Irons, 2004). This gave rise to two scales: 1. the forms of self-criticising/attacking and self-reassuring scale (FSCRS) and 2. the functions of self-criticising/attacking scale (FSCS). The FSCRS asks people how they think about themselves 'when things go wrong in our lives or don't work out as we hoped'. There were three clear factors. One was an ability to be self-reassuring and remind oneself of one's capabilities and past efforts. In regard to the self-critical items our factor analysis suggested two self-critical forms. One focused on a sense of disappointment and inadequacy while a second was more focused on self-hatred. Self-hatred turned out to be the more pathogenic, again highlighting the subtlety of important differences and function of these processes. The data suggested that you could be critical and disappointed with yourself but not hate yourself (maybe because you think you could or should be better), but self-hatred is different. Indeed, self-hatred was highly correlated with self-persecution and hurting the self ($r = .80$).

There is now a large literature on self-criticism measured with the scale, its relationship to processes such as perfectionism and a range of psychopathologies. A recent large meta-analysis confirmed a three factor solution which is stable and highly predictive of mental health problems (Halamová, Kanovský, Gilbert, Troop, Zuroff, Hermanto et al., 2018; Halamová, Kanovský, Gilbert, Troop, Zuroff, Petrocchi et al., 2018).

## A new focus for therapy: motivation switching and the role of caring motives

As the data on the competitive mentality and its role in mental health difficulties became stronger and stronger, our therapeutic interest switched more and more to how we could produce motivational shifts. In particular, how could we help people shift out of self-focused, competitive (and rank) motivational systems as ways of organising their self, and focus on sharing and caring? One of the reasons was because the physiological systems of these motivational systems are very different. In fact, over the last 20 years there has been considerable research looking at the complex physiological systems that underpin caring behaviour and the experience of being cared for. (For recent reviews see Gilbert (2017a) and Seppälä et al. (2017).)

One of the tasks was to develop an evolution and social mentality based approach to compassion, including its definition. Currently there are a number of variations, debates and controversies around compassion definitions (Gilbert, 2017b, 2017c). Most theorists interested in evolutionary approaches recognise that compassion evolved from mammalian caring behaviour, particularly maternal behaviour, where the stimulus (S) of the algorithm was some kind of distress or need signal, and the response function (R) was some kind of action to address need and/or alleviate stress. So compassion is rooted in mammalian motivational systems with an identified algorithm that leads to the definition of it being a 'sensitivity to suffering in self and others with a commitment to try to alleviate and prevent it' (Gilbert, 2017a). This algorithm also has identifiable physiological patterns and profiles linked to the frontal cortex, the evolution of the myelinated vagus nerve and hormones like oxytocin (Carter, Bartal, & Porge, 2017; Porges, 2017). Importantly the recipient of care, particularly the infant in the first instance, is highly physiologically regulated by caring, including brain maturation and even epigenetic processes (Cowan et al., 2016). Importantly these basic systems are also the ones that operate for adult caring.

However, there is more to compassion than just caring; otherwise all primates that care for their infants would be regarded as compassionate. It is our new brain competencies for certain types of thinking, forms of social intelligence, self-awareness and intentional behaviour that turn caring into compassion (Gilbert, 2017a). Indeed, these competencies change many types of motives. For example, the suffering a predator causes its prey is not regarded as sadistic or cruel because the predator has no intention of causing suffering; it acts to eat. In humans, however, we can have a deliberate intention to cause pain and suffering quite knowingly and in those circumstances we do call the behaviour cruel and sadistic. This is an example where it's the knowing, self and future aware – intentionality – of our behaviour that changes it. To sum up then we have algorithms which evolved with specific physiological profiles to enact and respond to caring behaviour. These can be triggered as antidotes to overly engaged self-focused competitive motives.

As part of our research endeavour we needed to develop measures of compassion and its inhibitors: what stops people from being compassionate to themselves or to others or receptive to the compassion from others. So our first scales were primarily fears of compassion because that was the therapeutic task (Gilbert, McEwan, Matos, & Rivis, 2011). The scales are being used internationally, resulting in a major meta-analysis which highlights the fact that fears of being compassionate to oneself and fears of being open to compassion from others is highly associated with mental health difficulties (Kirby, Day, & Sagar, 2019). It's also very clear that giving and receiving compassion are two quite different processes. Subsequently we developed scales to measure the three flows of compassion: compassion to self, openness to the compassion from others and compassion to others (Gilbert et al., 2017). These are now being used around the world. They have been contrasted with the more antisocial aspects of human behaviour (Basran et al., 2019).

## *Into the therapy*

Part of the impetus for recognising how essential it was to change motivational processing systems became apparent from working with one particularly chronically depressed person who had attempted suicide multiple times. She had had many years of different types of therapy including cognitive and psychodynamic and was competent at generating alternative thoughts to offset her sense of being unlovable and unwanted and as an adopted child. So I asked her to speak them out in exactly the way she heard them in her mind. It was a new Socratic question for me. The emotional tone of the thoughts was extremely bullying and aggressive even though the content was supportive. It was a bit of an eye-opener and I subsequently began to ask clients regularly to speak in the tone that they actually hear or create coping thoughts in their minds. If you could help clients overcome the embarrassment of saying exactly how they heard them, sure enough, coping thoughts were often hostile in emotional tone. In addition, clients acknowledged some irritation at having to try to monitor or write down their thoughts, although they wouldn't necessarily admit that to the therapist unless the therapist asked, 'How irritated might you feel that you have to monitor thoughts and then try to counteract them?'

Hence, the first movement of CFT was to help create compassion motivation and emotional tones to texture coping efforts. I would try to help the client get into a motivational state of wanting to be helpful to themselves. This proved to be much more difficult than anticipated, and I discovered many fears, blocks and resistances to moving into a compassionate, caring orientation for the self. Sometimes it was to do with the fact that being supportive and kind to oneself was just very unfamiliar and didn't seem real. Sometimes it opened up attachment difficulties that linked to neglectful or abusive experiences. Commonly, beginning to experience a 'kind-supportive' voice in one's head triggered overwhelming grief. When some chronically depressed individuals started to engage in compassion, they would touch a deep sense of loneliness they had carried for many years. The focusing on capacities for tolerating intense grief became a major element in CFT. Sometimes individuals had a lot of rage or shame about the past and indicated then that they didn't deserve compassion. Sometimes depressed people could be very hesitant to accept care or believe it. They tended to have views that people are caring only because it's in their interest to be caring, or if a caring person really knew about them, and what goes on in their mind, they would not be caring. Pauley and McPherson (2010) conducted a qualitative study that asked depressed people about being self-compassionate. It revealed many fears and inhibitors. Hence, as the therapy developed, it became clear that the therapist needed to work with the fears, blocks and resistances to compassion. So our next theme of research was to explore and measure the fears, blocks and resistances of compassion (see Kirby et al., 2019 for an overview of this research and meta-analysis on the measures).

## *The impact and legacy of the research and lessons learnt*

The last 40 years has shown that it's possible to take an evolutionary function analytic model and develop measures to tap into core evolved motivational systems and their regulators. It's very clear that humans pursue different strategies for their life tasks of survival and reproduction. Some are highly self-focused and competitive; others are much more caring and sharing. A combination of genes and early and later social contexts play their roles. Crucially, however, different motives and different strategies carry different vulnerabilities to mental health problems. As we began to understand the dark side of competition (Gilbert et al., 2009) it became more urgent to help people switch from being overly regulated through competitive psychologies to caring and sharing. This is not only to facilitate and buffer against mental health difficulties but also to promote prosocial and moral behaviour (See Gilbert & Mascaro, 2017 for an overview of the forms of inhibitors and see Kirby et al., 2019 for an overview of this research and meta-analysis on the measures).

## *Contrasting compassion with competition*

We now can contrast compassionate and competitive motivations in terms of how they orientate attention, focus our thinking, trigger emotions, choreograph our interpersonal behaviour with others around us and physiologically pattern our bodies.

Figure 1.2 shows that competitive psychology is focused on social ranks and one's position within these ranks: who to compare with, who

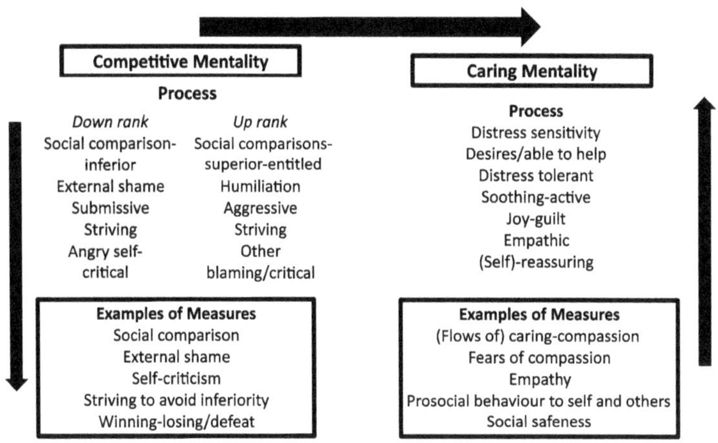


**FIGURE 1.2** Moving from a competitive to a caring social motive and mentality (copyright P. Gilbert)

can threaten or support us, who to associate with and who to impress. Individuals who are down-rank focused tend to be concerned with being inferior compared to others and are submissive and self-critical. As noted earlier there is now considerable evidence that depressed and socially anxious individuals are rank focused and concerned with their social attractiveness in the minds of others. These individuals also tend to be self-critical which can then give a sense of personal diminishment, shame, defeat and entrapment.

In contrast, individuals who are up-rank focused tend to be narcissistic with a sense of being relatively superior and entitled and have a tendency to blame others for difficulties. They can also be aggressive if confronted. There are many leaders in the world today who fit that latter category (Basran et al., 2019). For the most part these individuals do not present themselves for therapy because they often lack insight and are not that bothered about the distress they cause others. If they start to get anxious or depressed or run into addiction problems they might come to therapy. This is unfortunate because in a way it's precisely these individuals whom the rest of us would love to see getting some kind of therapy to help them change and become more compassionate!

Given that the competitive motivational system, with its focus on social rank, can underpin many psychological difficulties, what compassion training and compassion focused therapies try to do is to help people engage in motivational shifting. That is to shift attention, thinking and concerns from competitiveness into caring. There is a focus on developing insight into how caring and compassion focused mental states create more meaningful experiences in life, have major physiological impacts on well-being and create prosocial and supportive social contexts (Goleman & Davidson, 2017). A key focus is that compassion training can't simply focus on 'caring motives' without also recognising the other motivational systems that compete with them and often create the fears, blocks and resistances to compassion. Compassion will partly help offset other motivations when they become harmful. Part of the training is to target physiological systems such as the vagus nerve and frontal cortex by for example teaching breathing and postural exercises and using various visualizations that are designed to stimulate different physiological systems (Gilbert & Choden, 2013).

At the bottom of Figure 1.2 there is a note of some of the scales that this research endeavour has developed over the years. They enable opportunities to identify changes in the processes the scales measure as part of the therapeutic progress. It is well recognised that measures of change can't rely on self-report alone. Hence, compassion focused therapy is beginning to look in more detail at the physiological changes such as in heart rate variability and neurophysiological changes that can occur with compassion training. That's the next body of work – assuming one lives long enough!

## *Conclusion and personal observations*

Exploring the nature of the human mind requires considering how and why it got to be the way it is. This offers a functional analysis of what people need in order to prosper, flourish, buffer against mental health difficulties and behave morally and prosocially in the world. It's clear that humans are a multi-minded species of extremes; they can be both caring but also terrifyingly cruel to others and at times themselves, even to the point of self-hatred. Understanding the roots of these processes, as residing in the basic evolved motives and algorithms of the mind, is central for how to change them. In addition, understanding the social contextual shaping of these processes is key to move communities and nations to a more compassionate focus. Currently, it is well recognised that we are very vulnerable to instigating tribal conflicts with neoliberalism overly stimulating us to adopt competitive self-focused motives. Amongst the tragedy, trauma and chaos of COVID-19, faith in the market, narcissistic self-gratification and neoliberalism are fading. These do not provide the context to address many of the social ecological problems that we nor create the social conditions for wellbeing or do they reduce the high and increasing rates of mental health problems in our communities.

Understanding the conflict between competitive motives (that entice us to treat others as objects, to compare and rate ourselves, and develop fears of inferiority and exclusion) in contrast to compassion motives (that entice us to treat ourselves and others respectfully and 'carefully' as sentient beings) is therefore a crucial challenge for us. We have learnt, however, that switching people from competitive to compassion ways of living for both self and others is not always easy. Indeed, at times people can be fearful of, or highly resistant to, compassion. Addressing the inhibitors to compassion (Gilbert & Mascaro, 2017) maybe one of the processes that unleash a compassionate desire for all to flourish.

## References


Abbott, D. H., Keverne, E. B., Bercovitch, F. B., Shirely, C. A., Mendoza, S. P., Soltzman, W., . . . Sapolsky, R. M. (2004). Are subordinates always stressed? A comparative analysis of rank differences in cortisol levels among primates. *Hormones and Behavior, 43*, 67–82.

Akiskal, H. S., & McKinney, W. T. (1973). Depressive disorders: Toward a unified hypothesis. *Science, 182*, 20–29.

Allan, S., & Gilbert, P. (1995). A social comparison scale: Psychometric properties and relationship to psychopathology. *Personality and Individual Differences, 19*, 293–299.

Allan, S., & Gilbert, P. (1997). Submissive behaviour and psychopathology. *British Journal of Clinical Psychology, 36*, 467–488.

Allan, S., Gilbert, P., & Goss, K. (1994). An exploration of shame measures: II: Psychopathology. *Personality and Individual Differences, 17*, 719–722.

Anderson, C., Hildreth, J. A. D., & Howland, L. (2015). Is the desire for status a fundamental human motive? A review of the empirical literature. *Psychological Bulletin, 141*(3), 574.

Anderson, C., Kraus, M. W., Galinsky, A. D., & Keltner, D. (2012). The local-ladder effect: Social status and subjective well-being. *Psychological Science, 23*(7), 764–771.

Barkow, J. H. (1975). Prestige and culture: A biosocial interpretation (plus peer review). *Current Anthropology, 16*, 533–572.

Barrett, L. F. (2017). *How emotions are made: The secret life of the brain*. Boston, MA: Houghton Mifflin Harcourt.

Basran, J., Pires, C., Matos, M., McEwan, K., & Gilbert, P. (2019). Styles of leadership, fears of compassion, and competing to avoid inferiority. *Frontiers in Psychology, 9*, 2460. doi:10.3389/fpsyg.2018.02460

Bernard, C., Mills, M., Swenson, L., & Walsh, R. P. (2005). An evolutionary theory of human motivation. *Genetic, Social, and General Psychology Monographs, 131*, 129–184.

Birchwood, M., Meaden, A., Trower, P., Gilbert, P., & Plaistow, J. (2000). The power and omnipotence of voices: Subordination and entrapment by voices and significant others. *Psychological Medicine, 30*, 337–344.

Blizard, R. A. (2003). Disorganized attachment, development of dissociated self states, and a relational approach to treatment. *Journal of Trauma and Dissociation*, *4*, 27–50.

Boksem, M. A., Kostermans, E., Milivojevic, B., & De Cremer, D. (2011). Social status determines how we monitor and evaluate our performance. *Social Cognitive and Affective Neuroscience*, 7(3), 304–313.

Bowlby, J. (1969). *Attachment and loss, Vol. 1: Attachment*. London: Hogarth Press.

Bowlby, J. (1973). *Attachment and loss, Vol. 2: Separation, anxiety and anger*. London: Hogarth Press.

Bowlby, J. (1980). *Attachment and loss, Vol. 3: Sadness and depression – attachment and loss*. London: Hogarth Press.

Brown, G. W., & Harris, T. O. (1978). *The social origins of depression*. London: Tavistock.

Brown, G. W., Harris, T. O., & Hepworth, C. (1995). Loss, humiliation and entrapment among women developing depression: A patient and non-patient comparison. *Psychological Medicine*, *25*, 7–21.

Brugha, T. (1995). *Social support & psychiatric disorder: Research findings and guidelines for clinical practice*. Cambridge: Cambridge University Press.

Brüne, M. (2015). *Textbook of evolutionary psychiatry and psychosomatic medicine: The origins of psychopathology*. Oxford: Oxford University Press.

Buss, D. M. (2015). *Evolutionary psychology: The new science of the mind*. New York, NY: Psychology Press.

Buss, D. M., & Craik, K. H. (1986). Acts, dispositions and clinical assessments: The psychopathology of everyday contact. *Clinical Psychology Review*, *6*, 387–406.

Carter, S., Bartal, I. B., & Porges, E. (2017). The roots of compassion: An evolutionary and neurobiological perspective. In E. M. Seppälä, E. Simon-Thomas, S. L. Brown, & M. C. Worline (Eds.), *The Oxford handbook of compassion science* (pp. 178–188). New York, NY: Oxford University Press.

Carvalho, S., Pinto-Gouveia, J., Pimentel, P., Maia, D., Gilbert, P., & Mota-Pereira, J. (2013). Entrapment and defeat perceptions in depressive symptomatology: Through an evolutionary approach. *Psychiatry: Interpersonal & Biological Processes*, *76*(1), 53–67.

Cassidy, J., & Shaver, P. R. (2016). *Handbook of attachment: Theory, research and clinical applications* (3rd ed.). New York, NY: Guilford Press.

Chua, K. J., Lukaszewski, A. W., Grant, D. M., & Sng, O. (2016). Human life history strategies: Calibrated to external or internal cues? *Evolutionary Psychology*, *15*(1). doi:1474704916677342

Clarke, M., McEwan, K., Ness, J., Waters, K., Basran, J., & Gilbert, P. (2016). A descriptive study of feelings of arrested escape (entrapment) and arrested anger in people presenting to an emergency department following an episode of self-harm. *Frontiers in Psychiatry*, 7, 155.

Cooley, C. H. (1902). Looking-glass self. In *The production of reality: Essays and readings on social interaction* (6th ed.). Los Angeles, CA: University of California Press.

Cowan, C. S. M., Callaghan, B. L., Kan, J. M., & Richardson, R. (2016). The lasting impact of early-life adversity on individuals and their descendants: Potential mechanisms and hope for intervention. *Genes, Brain and Behavior, 15*(1), 155–168.

Crawford, C., & Krebs, D. L. (2013). *Handbook of evolutionary psychology: Ideas, issues, and applications*. New York, NY: Psychology Press.

Curran, T., & Hill, A. P. (2019). Perfectionism is increasing over time: A meta-analysis of birth cohort differences from 1989 to 2016. *Psychological Bulletin, 145*, 410–425.

Del Giudice, M. (2016). The life history model of psychopathology explains the structure of psychiatric disorders and the emergence of the p factor: A simulation study. *Clinical Psychological Science, 4*, 299–311. Retrieved from https://doi.org/10.1177/2167702615583628

Dixon, A. K. (1998). Ethological strategies for defence in animals and humans: Their role in some psychiatric disorders. *British Journal of Medical Psychology, 71*, 417–445.

Dixon, A. K., Fisch, H. U., Huber, C., & Walser, A. (1989). Ethological studies in animals and man: Their use of psychiatry. *Pharmacopsychiatry, 22*, 44–50. doi:10.1055/s-2007-1014624

Dunbar, R. I. M. (2017). *Human evolution: A pelican introduction*. London: Penguin.

Dunbar, R. I. M., & Barrett, L. (2007). *The Oxford handbook of evolutionary psychology*. Oxford: Oxford University Press.

Ellenberger, H. F. (1970). *The discovery of the unconscious: The history and evolution of dynamic psychiatry*. New York, NY: Basic Books.

Fournier, M. A., Moskowitz, D. S., & Zuroff, D. C. (2002). Social rank strategies in hierarchical relationships. *Journal of Personality and Social Psychology, 83*, 425–433.

Freud, S. (1917). Mourning and melancholia. In J. Strachey (Ed. & Trans.), *Completed psychological works* (Vol. 14, Standard ed.). London: Hogarth Press.

Gilbert, P. (1980). *An investigation of cognitive factors and depression*. PhD Thesis, University of Edinburgh.

Gilbert, P. (1984). *Depression: From psychology to brain state*. London: Lawrence Erlbaum Associates.

Gilbert, P. (1988). Psychobiological interactions in depression. In S. Fisher & J. Reason (Eds.), *Handbook of life stress, cognition and health* (pp. 559–579). Chichester: Wiley.

Gilbert, P. (1989). *Human nature and suffering* (p. 406). London: Lawrence Erlbaum Associates.

Gilbert, P. (1992). *Depression: The evolution of powerlessness*. London: Lawrence Erlbaum Associates.

Gilbert, P. (1995). Biopsychosocial approaches and evolutionary theory as aids to integration in clinical psychology and psychotherapy. *Clinical Psychology and Psychotherapy, 2*, 135–156.

Gilbert, P. (1997). The evolution of social attractiveness and its role in shame, humiliation, guilt and therapy. *British Journal of Medical Psychology, 70*, 113–147.

Gilbert, P. (1998). Evolutionary psychopathology: Why isn't the mind better designed than it is? *British Journal of Medical Psychology*, *71*, 353–373.

Gilbert, P. (2000). Varieties of submissive behaviour: Their evolution and role in depression. In L. Sloman & P. Gilbert (Eds.), *Subordination and defeat: An evolutionary approach to mood disorders* (pp. 3–46). Hillsdale, NJ: Lawrence Erlbaum Associates.

Gilbert, P. (2001). Evolutionary approaches to psychopathology: The role of natural defences. *Australian and New Zealand Journal of Psychiatry*, *35*, 17–27.

Gilbert, P. (2006). Evolution and depression: Issues and implications (invited review). *Psychological Medicine*, *36*, 287–297.

Gilbert, P. (2007). *Psychotherapy and counselling for depression* (3rd ed.). London: Sage.

Gilbert, P. (2013). Depression: The challenges of an integrated, biopsychosocial evolutionary approach. In M. Power (Ed.), *The Wiley Blackwell handbook of mood disorders: Second edition* (pp. 229–288). Chichester: Wiley.

Gilbert, P. (2016). A biopsychosocial and evolutionary approach to formulation. In N. Tarrier (Ed.), *Case formulation in cognitive behaviour therapy: The treatment of challenging cases* (2nd ed., pp. 50–89). Chichester: Wiley.

Gilbert, P. (2017a). Compassion as a social mentality: An evolutionary approach. In P. Gilbert (Ed.), *Compassion: Concepts, research and applications* (pp. 31–68). London: Routledge.

Gilbert, P. (2017b). Compassion: Definitions and controversies. In P. Gilbert (Ed.), *Compassion: Concepts, research and applications* (pp. 3–15). London: Routledge.

Gilbert, P. (Ed.). (2017c). *Compassion: Concepts, research and applications* (pp. 3–15). London: Routledge.

Gilbert, P. (2018). *Living like crazy* (2nd ed.). York: Annwyn House.

Gilbert, P. (2019a). Psychotherapy for the 21st century: An integrative, evolutionary, contextual, biopsychosocial approach. *Psychology and Psychotherapy: Theory, Research and Practice*, *92*, 164–189.

Gilbert, P. (2019b). Distinguishing shame, humiliation and guilt: An evolutionary functional analysis and compassion focused interventions. In C.-H. Mayer & E. Vanderheiden (Eds.), *The bright side of shame* (pp. 413–432). New York, NY: Springer.

Gilbert, P., & Allan, S. (1994). Assertiveness, submissive behaviour and social comparison. *British Journal of Clinical Psychology*, *33*, 295–306.

Gilbert, P., & Allan, S. (1998). The role of defeat and entrapment (arrested flight) in depression: An exploration of an evolutionary view. *Psychological Medicine*, *28*, 584–597.

Gilbert, P., Allan, S., Brough, S., Melly, S., & Miles, J. N.V. (2002). Relationship of anhenoia and anxiety to social rank, defeat and entrapment. *Journal of Affective Disorders*, *71*, 141–151.

Gilbert, P., Birchwood, M., Gilbert, J., Trower, P., Hay, J., Murray, B., . . . Miles, J. N. V. (2001). An exploration of evolved mental mechanisms for dominant and subordinate behaviour in relation to auditory hallucinations in schizophrenia and critical thoughts in depression. *Psychological Medicine*, *31*, 1117–1127.

Gilbert, P., Broomhead, C., Irons, C., McEwan, K., Bellew, R., Mills, A., & Gale, C. (2007). Striving to avoid inferiority: Scale development and its relationship to depression, anxiety and stress. *British Journal of Social Psychology*, *46*, 633–648.

Gilbert, P., Catarino, F., Duarte, C., Matos, M., Kolts, R., Stubbs, J., . . . Basran, J. (2017). The development of compassionate engagement and action scales for self and others. *Journal of Compassionate Health Care*, *4*(1), 1–24. doi:10.1186/s40639-017-0033-3

Gilbert, P., & Choden, K. (2013). *Mindful compassion*. London: Little Brown.

Gilbert, P., Clarke, M., Kempel, S., Miles, J. N.V., & Irons, C. (2004). Criticizing and reassuring oneself: An exploration of forms style and reasons in female students. *British Journal of Clinical Psychology*, *43*, 31–50.

Gilbert, P., Gilbert, J., & Irons, C. (2004). Life events, entrapments and arrested anger in depression. *Journal of Affective Disorders*, *79*(1–3), 149–160.

Gilbert, P., & Irons, C. (2005). Focused therapies and compassionate mind training for shame and self-attacking. In P. Gilbert (Ed.), *Compassion: Conceptualisations, research and use in psychotherapy* (pp. 263–325). London: Routledge.

Gilbert, P & Mascaro, J. (2017). Compassion: Fears, blocks, and resistances: An evolutionary investigation. In, Seppälä, E.M., Simon-Thomas, E., Brown, S.L., Worline, M.C., Cameron, L & Doty, J. R. (Eds). *The Oxford Handbook of Compassion Science*. (pp. 399–420). New York: Oxford University Press.

Gilbert, P., McEwan, K., Irons, C., Broomhead, C., Bellew, R., Mills, A., & Gale, C. (2009). The dark side of competition: How competitive behaviour and striving to avoid inferiority, are linked to depression, anxiety, stress and self-harm. *Psychology and Psychotherapy*, *82*, 123–136.

Gilbert, P., McEwan, K., Matos, M., & Rivis, A. (2011). Fears of compassion: Development of three self-report measures. *Psychology and Psychotherapy*, *84*(3), 239–255. doi:10.1348/147608310X526511

Gilbert, P., & Miles, J. N.V. (2000). Sensitivity to put down: Its relationship to perceptions of shame, social anxiety, depression, anger and self-other blame. *Personality and Individual Differences*, *29*, 757–774.

Gilbert, P., Price, J. S., & Allan, S. (1995). Social comparison, social attractiveness and evolution: How might they be related? *New Ideas in Psychology*, *13*, 149–165.

Goleman, D., & Davidson, R. J. (2017). *Altered traits: Science reveals how meditation changes your mind, brain, and body*. London: Penguin.

Goss, K., Gilbert, P., & Allan, S. (1994). An exploration of shame measures: I: The 'other as shamer' scale. *Personality and Individual Differences*, *17*, 713–717.

Grewen, K. M., Girdler, S. S., Amico, J., & Light, K. C. (2005). Effects of partner support on resting oxytocin, cortisol, norepinephrine, and blood pressure before and after warm partner contact. *Psychosomatic Medicine*, *67*(4), 531–538.

Griffiths, A. W., Wood, A. M., Maltby, J., Taylor, P. J., & Tai, S. (2014). The prospective role of defeat and entrapment in depression and anxiety: A 12-month longitudinal study. *Psychiatry Research*, *216*(1), 52–59.

Griffiths, A. W., Wood, A. M., & Tai, S. (2018). The prospective role of defeat and entrapment in caregiver burden and depression amongst formal caregivers. *Personality and Individual Differences*, *120*, 24–31.

Halamová, J., Kanovský, M., Gilbert, P., Troop, N. A., Zuroff, D. C., Hermanto, N., . . . Kupeli, N. (2018). The factor structure of the forms of self-criticising/attacking & self-reassuring scale in thirteen distinct populations. *Journal of Psychopathology and Behavioral Assessment*, 1–16.

Halamová, J., Kanovský, M., Gilbert, P., Troop, N. A., Zuroff, D. C., Petrocchi, N., . . . Kupeli, N. (2018). Multiple group IRT measurement invariance: Analysis of the forms of self-criticising/attacking and self-reassuring scale in thirteen international samples. *Journal of Rational Emotive and Cognitive Behaviour Therapy*. Retrieved from doi.org/10.1007/s10942-019-00319-1

Heinrichs, M., Baumgartner, T., Kirschbaum, C., & Ehlert, U. (2003). Social support and oxytocin interact to suppress cortisol and subjective responses to psychosocial stress. *Biological Psychiatry, 54*(12), 1389–1398.

Higley, J. D., Mehlman, P. T., Higley, S., Fremald, B., Vickers, J., Lindell, S. G., . . . Linnoila, M. (1996). Excessive mortality in young free-ranging male nonhuman primates with low cerebrospinal fluid 5-hydroxyindoleacetic acid concentrations. *Archives of General Psychiatry, 53*, 537–543.

Hill, D. (1968). Depression: Disease, reaction or posture? *American Journal of Psychiatry, 125*, 445-457.

Höller, I., Teismann, T., Cwik, J. C., Glaesmer, H., Spangenberg, L., Hallensleben, N., . . . Forkmann, T. (2020). Short defeat and entrapment scale: A psychometric investigation in three German samples. *Comprehensive Psychiatry*, 152160.

Kannan, D., & Levitt, H. M. (2013). A review of client self-criticism in psychotherapy. *Journal of Psychotherapy Integration, 23*(2), 166.

Kelly, A. C., Zuroff, D. C., Leybman, M. J., & Gilbert, P. (2012). Social safeness, received social support, and maladjustment: Testing a tripartite model of affect regulation. *Cognitive Therapy and Research, 36*, 815–826. doi:10.1007/s10608–011–9432

Kim, S., Thibodeau, R., & Jorgensen, R. S. (2011). Shame, guilt, and depressive symptoms: A meta-analytic review. *Psychological Bulletin, 137*, 68–96. doi:10.1037/a0021466

Kirby, J. N., Day, J., & Sagar, V. (2019). The 'flow' of compassion: A meta-analysis of the fears of compassion scales and psychological functioning. *Clinical Psychology Review, 70*, 26–39.

Liotti, G. (2000). Disorganised attachment, models of borderline states and evolutionary psychotherapy. In P. Gilbert & K. G. Bailey (Eds.), *Genes on the couch explorations and evolutionary psychotherapy* (pp. 232–256). London: Routledge.

Longe, O., Maratos, F. A., Gilbert, P., Evans, G., Volker, F., Rockliffe, H., & Rippon, G. (2010). Having a word with yourself: Neural correlates of self-criticism and self-reassurance. *NeuroImage, 49*, 1849–1856.

Marsh, A. A. (2019). The caring continuum: Evolved hormonal and proximal mechanisms explain prosocial and antisocial extremes. *Annual Review of Psychology, 70*, 347–371.

McEwan, K., Gilbert, P., & Duarte, J. (2012). An exploration of competitiveness and caring in relation to psychopathology. *British Journal of Clinical Psychology, 51*, 19–36. doi:10.1111/j.2044-8260.2011.02010.x

McGuire, M.T., & Troisi, A. (1998). *Darwinian psychiatry*. New York, NY: Oxford University Press.

Music, G. (2019). *Nurturing natures' attachment and children's emotional sociocultural and brain development* (2nd ed.). London: Routledge.

Nesse, R. M. (2000). Is depression an adaptation? *Archives of General Psychiatry*, *57*, 14–20.

Nesse, R. M. (2019). *Good reasons for bad feelings: Insights from the frontier of evolutionary psychiatry*. New York, NY: Dutton.

Nesse, R. M., & Williams, G. C. (1995). *Evolution & healing*. London: Weidenfeld & Nicolson.

Panksepp, J. (1998). *Affective neuroscience: The foundations of human and animal emotions*. New York, NY: Oxford University Press.

Pauley, G., & McPherson, S. (2010). The experience and meaning of compassion and self-compassion for individuals with depression or anxiety. *Psychology and Psychotherapy: Theory, Research and Practice*, *83*(2), 129–143.

Peterson, C., Maier, S. F., & Seligman, M. E. P. (1993). *Learned helplessness: A theory for the age of personal control*. New York, NY: Oxford University Press.

Petrocchi, N., & Cheli, S. (2019). The social brain and heart rate variability: Implications for psychotherapy. *Psychology and Psychotherapy: Theory, Research and Practice*, *92*(2), 208–223.

Porges, S. W. (2017). Vagal pathways: Portals to compassion. In E. M. Seppälä, E. Simon-Thomas, S. L. Brown, & M. C. Worline (Eds.), *The Oxford handbook of compassion science*. New York, NY: Oxford University Press.

Price, J. S. (1972). Genetic and phylogenetic aspects of mood variations. *International Journal of Mental Health*, *1*, 124-144.

Price, J. S. (2000). Subordination, self-esteem, and depression. In L. Sloman & P. Gilbert (Eds.), *Subordination and defeat: An evolutionary approach to mood disorders and their therapy* (pp. 165–177). Mahwah, NJ: Lawrence Erlbaum Associates.

Price, J. S., & Sloman, L. (1987). Depression as yielding behaviour: An animal model based on Schjelderup-Ebb's pecking order. *Ethology and Sociobiology*, *8*(Supplement), 85-98.

Price, J. S., Sloman, L., Gardner, R., Gilbert, P., & Rohde, P. (1994). The social competition hypothesis of depression. *British Journal of Psychiatry*, *164*, 309–315.

Ryan, C. (2019). *Civilised to death: The price of progress*. London: Simon & Schuster.

Sapolsky, M. R. (2017). *Behave: The biology of humans at our best and worst*. London: Vintage.

Seligman, M. E. P. (1975). *Helplessness: On depression development and death*. San Francisco, CA: Freeman & Co.

Selten, J. P., van der Ven, E., Rutten, B. P., & Cantor-Graae, E. (2013). The social defeat hypothesis of schizophrenia: An update. *Schizophrenia Bulletin*, *39*(6), 1180–1186.

Selye, H. (1936). A syndrome produced by diverse nocuous agents. *Nature*, *138*, 32.

Seppälä, E. M., Simon-Thomas, E., Brown, S. L., Worline, M. C., Cameron, C. D., & Doty, J. R. (Eds.). (2017). *The Oxford handbook of compassion science*. New York, NY: Oxford University Press.

Siddaway, A. P., Taylor, P. J., Wood, A. M., & Schulz, J. (2015). A meta-analysis of perceptions of defeat and entrapment in depression, anxiety problems, posttraumatic stress disorder, and suicidality. *Journal of Affective Disorders*, *184*, 149–159.

Sloman, L. (2000). The syndrome of rejection sensitivity: An evolutionary perspective. In P. Gilbert (Ed.), *Genes on the couch* (pp. 257–275). London: Routledge.

Sloman, L., & Gilbert, P. (2000). *Subordination and defeat: An evolutionary approach to mood disorders*. Mahwah, NJ: Lawrence Erlbaum Associates.

Sturman, E. D., & Mongrain, M. (2005). Self-criticism and major depression: An evolutionary perspective. *British Journal of Clinical Psychology*, *44*, 505–519.

Sturman, E. D., Rose, S., McKeighan, K. M., Burch, J., & Evanico, K. (2015). Personality and the generation of defeat, involuntary subordination, and depression. *Canadian Journal of Behavioural Science/Revue canadienne des sciences du comportement*, *47*(1), 47.

Sznycer, D., Xygalatas, D., Agey, E., Alami, S., An, X. F., Ananyeva, K. I., . . . Fukushima, S. (2018). Cross-cultural invariances in the architecture of shame. *Proceedings of the National Academy of Sciences*, *115*(39), 9702–9707.

Taylor, P. J., Gooding, P., Wood, A. M., & Tarrier, N. (2011). The role of defeat and entrapment in depression, anxiety, and suicide. *Psychological Bulletin*, *137*(3), 391–420.

Taylor, P., Wood, A. M., Gooding, P., Johnson, J., & Tarrier, N. (2009). Are defeat and entrapment best defined as a single construct? *Personality and Individual Differences*, *47*, 795–797.

Valmaggia, L. R., Day, F., Garety, P., Freeman, D., Antley, A., Slater, M., . . . McGuire, P. (2015). Social defeat predicts paranoid appraisals in people at high risk for psychosis. *Schizophrenia Research*, *168*(1–2), 16–22.

Weiss, J. M., Demetrikopoulos, M. K., McCurdy, P. M., West, C. H. K., & Bonsall, R. W. (2000). Depression seen through an animal model: An expanded hypothesis of pathophysiology and improved models. In R. J. Davidson (Ed.), *Anxiety, depression and emotion* (pp. 3–35). New York, NY: Oxford University Press.

Wetherall, K., Robb, K. A., & O'Connor, R. C. (2019). Social rank theory of depression: A systematic review of self-perceptions of social rank and their relationship with depressive symptoms and suicide risk. *Journal of Affective Disorders*, *246*, 30–39. Retrieved from https://doi.org/10.1016/j.jad.2018.12.045

Whelton, W. J., & Greenberg, L. S. (2005). Emotion in self-criticism. *Personality and Individual Differences*, *38*, 1583–1595.

World Health Organisation. (2018). *Depression*. Retrieved from www.who.int/news-room/fact-sheets/detail/depression

Zeigler-Hill, V., Welling, L. L., & Shackelford, T. K. (Eds.). (2015). *Evolutionary perspectives on social psychology*. New York, NY: Springer.

# 2

# THE INFLUENCE OF ATTACHMENTS IN CLOSE RELATIONSHIPS ON MENTAL HEALTH

*Christopher A. Pepping and Geoff MacDonald*

The evolution of attachment behaviour between parent and infant is now recognized to be a template for adult relating in humans (Cassidy & Shaver, 2016; Fletcher, Simpson, Campbell, & Overall, 2015; Fisher, Aron, & Brown, 2006). In the transition from childhood to adulthood people transfer their attachment needs to peers and sexual partners, especially those who may form the basis of longer term relating and reproducing (Holmes, 2001). Here we present an overview of our own research, and that of others, pertaining to relationships and mental health from an attachment perspective. We begin with a review of the mental health benefits associated with satisfying romantic relationships. Next, we provide an overview of attachment theory and the relevance of adult attachment theory for understanding romantic relationships. We then present some of our recent work on attachment and long-term singlehood, and discuss the potential mental health implications of singlehood.

## Romantic relationships are protective

A satisfying romantic relationship serves many functions relating to offering a secure base, emotion regulation, and supporting self-esteem. Married individuals report higher well-being and happiness compared to those who are unmarried, divorced, or widowed (Diener, Suh, Lucas, & Smith, 1999; Lucas & Dyrenforth, 2005). A recent meta-analysis reveals that being in a satisfying romantic relationship is associated with greater physical health and lower mortality (Robles, Slatcher, Trombello, & McGinn, 2014). In contrast, those who are long-term single report elevated depression and anxiety and less sexual satisfaction (Schachner, Shaver, & Gillath, 2008).

The association between relationship status and mental health outcomes is complex. Some have argued that the marriage benefit is overstated and data do not support the widespread claims of increased well-being for married individuals (DePaulo & Morris, 2005). Indeed, associations between marital status and well-being are often small, vary across nations, and some studies have compared only currently satisfied couples with all non-married individuals, including those who are divorced, which itself can be associated with low well-being for some people (Kurdek, 1991; Lucas & Dyrenforth, 2005; Sbarra, Hasselmo, & Bourassa, 2015). Nonetheless, Lucas and Dyrenforth (2005) analyzed data from the World Values Survey, a multi-national study of approximately 170,000 people from more than 70 nations, and calculated effect size differences in life satisfaction between married and never-married individuals across three time points. The strength and direction of the association between marital status and well-being varied across nations, though in the USA, married individuals had consistently higher life satisfaction compared to those who had never married ($d$ = .30–.47).

We suggest that simply comparing coupled and single individuals on indices of well-being does not capture the diversity *within* these two groups. For instance, the benefits of relationships result from being in a *satisfying* relationship whereas relationship distress is associated with elevated risk for a range of mental health problems (Whisman, 2007). Similarly, those who are satisfied being single report higher well-being than those who are less satisfied with singlehood (Lehmann et al., 2015). This heterogeneity has important implications for public policy and intervention development. Specifically, the research suggesting that single individuals fare worse than their coupled counterparts would have quite different policy implications to those suggested by the work of DePaulo and colleagues (e.g., DePaulo & Morris, 2005) who argue that the benefit of coupledom is overstated. Thus, we suggest that an individual difference perspective may provide clarity here. Attachment theory has proven to be one of the most productive frameworks for conceptualizing and understanding relationship processes in adulthood (Cassidy & Shaver, 2016; Mikulincer & Shaver, 2016). We now provide a brief overview of attachment theory, and then outline how attachment theory may be a useful framework for conceptualizing singlehood and associated mental health outcomes.

## Adult attachment theory and romantic relationships

Attachment theory (Bowlby, 1969, 1973, 1980) posits that humans have a biologically evolved attachment system that motivates infants to maintain proximity to attachment figures (usually parents during childhood) as it increases the chances of human survival. The function of the attachment system is to protect infants from physical and psychological harm, and to facilitate the development of emotion regulation, enabling them to confidently explore the world and participate in social relationships (Bowlby, 1969; Mikulincer & Shaver, 2016). Attachment figures serve three important functions: (1) they are targets for proximity seeking, (2) they function as a safe haven when an infant is distressed or in need, and (3) they act as a secure base from which an infant can confidently pursue other goals (Mikulincer & Shaver, 2016).

There are individual differences in attachment-system functioning that attachment theory argues develop based on repeated experiences with attachment figures. When caregivers are sensitive and responsive to infants' needs, infants typically develop a secure attachment style and experience "felt security – a sense that the world is generally safe, that attachment figures are helpful when called upon, and that it is possible to explore the environment curiously and confidently and to engage rewardingly with other people" (Mikulincer & Shaver, 2007, p. 21). In the absence of such sensitivity and responsiveness, infants adopt secondary attachment strategies. Inconsistent responsiveness results in *hyperactivation* of the attachment system; infants intensify proximity seeking behaviours and do not give up easily as they sometimes succeed in gaining proximity (Main, 1990; Mikulincer & Shaver, 2016). Attachment system *deactivation* results from attachment figures being consistently unavailable, rejecting, and punitive of proximity seeking. Deactivation is characterized by suppression of attachment needs and decreased bids for proximity to keep the attachment system down-regulated, thus preventing disappointment associated with unresponsive attachment figures (Main, 1990; Mikulincer & Shaver, 2016).

Attachment in adulthood tends to be conceptualized along the two dimensions of attachment anxiety (attachment system hyperactivation) and attachment avoidance (attachment system deactivation). Attachment anxiety is characterized by sensitivity to rejection and abandonment, fear that support from attachment figures will not be provided, and anger and distress when attachment needs are not met (Fraley, Waller, & Brennan, 2000; Mikulincer & Shaver, 2016). In contrast, those high in attachment avoidance keep the attachment system down-regulated, are uncomfortable with intimacy and closeness, deny emotional vulnerability, and are excessively self-reliant (Fraley et al., 2000; Mikulincer & Shaver, 2016). People who are low in attachment anxiety and avoidance have an internal working model, or script, of attachment security.

Over 30 years of research demonstrates that adult attachment security is associated with stable and satisfying romantic relationships, whereas attachment insecurity (anxiety and avoidance) is associated with poor relationship outcomes (Mikulincer & Shaver, 2016). For instance, attachment insecurity is associated with low relationship satisfaction in established couples, and predicts relationship instability (Mikulincer & Shaver, 2012), shorter relationship duration (Hazan & Shaver, 1987), and higher rates of relationship break-up (Kirkpatrick & Hazan, 1994). As mentioned earlier, the quality of one's romantic relationship is a strong predictor of mental health and well-being. Attachment research has typically focused on the implications of adult attachment for established relationships. However, given that attachment orientations are internalized representations of relationship experiences that can be activated regardless of relationship status, our recent work has focused on the application of attachment theory for understanding long-term singlehood. An individual difference perspective on singlehood is likely to assist in understanding the variation in well-being within this heterogeneous group, and will also allow for the development of targeted policy and intervention. We now turn to our recent work on attachment and singlehood.

## Attachment and singlehood: implications for mental health

Rates of singlehood are rapidly increasing in Western countries. For instance, in the United States, approximately 28% of the adult population was single in 1970 (never married, divorced, or widowed), and this figure had risen to about 44% by 2010. Similar trends have been found in other Western countries such as England and Wales (Office for National Statistics, 2019), Canada (Statistics Canada, 2015) and Australia (Australian Institute of Family Studies, 2019), at least among opposite-sex couples. Clearly, a portion of this increase can be accounted for by increased cohabitation outside of marriage; however, this accounts for a reasonably small proportion of single people, and more people now live alone compared to any other point in history (U.S. Census Bureau, 1970, 2011, 2017). Singles are a sizeable and growing group of individuals, yet psychological research has largely ignored the topic of singlehood. Our recent work has focused on understanding singlehood from an attachment perspective (Pepping & MacDonald, 2019; Pepping, MacDonald, & Davis, 2018).

In recognition of the rise in singlehood, early sociological work began to ask the question of why some people remain long-term single (e.g., Forsyth & Johnson, 1995; Stein, 1978). These early theoretical reviews posited that long-term singles are likely to be a heterogeneous group of people. For some it may represent a personal desire to remain single, whereas for others it may reflect difficulties in establishing or maintaining romantic relationships (Keith, 1980; Stein, 1978). Indeed, qualitative research tends to support this proposition. Forsyth and Johnson (1995) conducted structured interviews with 204 adults over 35 who had never married, and asked participants the reasons they had not married. Only 23 individuals (11%) reported not wanting to marry, and 102 (50%) stated they had not met the right person. Other reasons included excessive work commitments and previous negative experiences in relationships. A qualitative study of 16 individuals (eight men and eight women) aged between 62 and 87 who had never married found varied reasons for remaining single (Band-Winterstein & Manchik-Rimon, 2014). For some it was a personal choice, and entering a romantic relationship was not an important goal; others attributed being single to having to care for elderly parents, previous experiences of being hurt in a relationship, and comparing potential partners with a lost love. In brief, there is increasing evidence that suggests long-term singles are a heterogeneous group (e.g., Band-Winterstein & Manchik-Rimon, 2014; Forsyth & Johnson, 1995).

Remarkably little psychological research has examined predictors of singlehood that might help us make sense of this heterogeneity. The few studies that have addressed such questions have used attachment theory as a theoretical framework. Schachner and colleagues (2008) compared a sample (*M* age = 40) of 73 coupled and 69 long-term single individuals (defined as single for the past three years, and unlikely to enter a romantic relationship in the next year) on the quality of their relationships with their parents during childhood, and adult attachment. Long-term singles reported more difficult relationships with their parents during childhood, but no significant differences in attachment were found between singles and couples. Specifically, although attachment anxiety (*d* = .26) and avoidance (*d* = .23) were somewhat higher in the group of long-term singles, these differences were not statistically significant.

In our own research, we recruited a US sample of 400 long-term single individuals, defined as not being in a committed romantic relationship for the past three years or more, and 407 individuals currently in a romantic relationship of at least one-year duration (Ringstad & Pepping, 2016). Long-term single individuals were higher in attachment anxiety (*d* = .32) and attachment avoidance (*d* = 1.01) compared to their partnered counterparts. Several other studies have addressed similar questions (e.g., Adamczyk & Bookwala, 2013; Petrowski, Schurig, Schmutzer, Brahler, & Stobel-Richter, 2015). These studies suggest that attachment insecurity does seem to be associated with single status, though there are discrepancies between studies in terms of which specific dimensions of attachment predict singlehood, and the strength of these associations (see Pepping et al., 2018 for a review).

We have argued that long-term singles are a heterogeneous group (Pepping et al., 2018), and the limited available evidence tends to support this proposition (e.g., Forsyth & Johnson, 1995; Band-Winterstein & Manchik-Rimon, 2014). In other words, there are likely to be multiple pathways to long-term singlehood; for some it may reflect underlying anxiety about relationships and difficulties forming stable relationships (consistent with high attachment anxiety), whereas for others it may reflect discomfort with intimacy and closeness (consistent with high attachment avoidance). Still for others, singlehood may be a personal choice whereby an individual's attachment needs are met outside of committed romantic relationships and may not, therefore, reflect attachment insecurity. Thus, simply comparing singles with those currently in a committed relationship is unlikely to fully capture the diverse nature of this population. This heterogeneity may well explain the inconsistencies in the literature, particularly if recruitment methods vary across studies and are tapping different sub-groups of singles.

In our recent work, we outlined distinct sub-groups of singles based on attachment theory (Pepping & MacDonald, 2019; Pepping et al., 2018). Here we outline our attachment theoretical model of long-term singlehood, including evidence suggestive of distinct sub-groups of singles: (1) singlehood due to attachment avoidance, (2) singlehood due to attachment anxiety, and (3) singlehood as a secure personal choice. We then describe the potential mental health and well-being outcomes for the three sub-groups.

## Avoidant attachment and singlehood

Those who are high in attachment avoidance possess a unique constellation of cognitive, affective, and behavioural characteristics that undermine the potential for intimacy and closeness. Avoidant individuals have experienced significant others to be unavailable when called upon, and thus they maintain attachment system deactivation to reduce the vulnerability that comes with seeking intimacy and closeness (Mikulincer & Shaver, 2016). Research from our own labs suggests that avoidant individuals tend to perceive less opportunity for intimacy in relationships, especially when there is a reasonable possibility for connection (Spielmann, Maxwell, MacDonald, & Baratta, 2013). Interestingly, when asked to consider a hypothetical renewal of their relationship with an ex-partner (who they had previously indicated they were unlikely to pursue), attachment avoidance was not associated with reduced expectations for intimacy and closeness. Thus, when there is an opportunity for connection, avoidant individuals appear to have a defence activated that keeps their hopes for intimacy low in order to prevent attachment system activation, and thereby avoid the vulnerability associated with potential rejection or disappointment.

Avoidant attachment decreases the likelihood a committed romantic relationship will develop. Commitment develops as partners become increasingly dependent on one another, which is diametrically opposed to the deactivating strategy designed to reduce dependence on others (Mikulincer & Shaver, 2016). Accordingly, those high in attachment avoidance express reduced commitment in romantic relationships, and are more likely to be on the lookout for potential alternative partners (Quirk et al., 2015). Qualitative studies suggest one reason for long-term singlehood is prior negative experiences in relationships (Band-Winterstein & Manchik-Rimon, 2014; Forsyth & Johnson, 1995). Individuals high in attachment avoidance are less likely to look for a new romantic partner following a break-up and, irrespective of whether the break-up was self-initiated or partner initiated, attachment avoidance is associated with avoiding potential new relationships (Davis, Shaver, & Vernon, 2003). Thus, attachment avoidance may prevent the formation of romantic relationships following prior relationship break-up, which is consistent with qualitative research revealing that some long-term singles report remaining single due to past experiences of being hurt in relationships (e.g., Band-Winterstein & Manchik-Rimon, 2014; Forsyth & Johnson, 1995).

Attachment system deactivation also undermines sexual intimacy. Attachment avoidance is associated with reduced frequency of sex (Bogaert & Sadava, 2002), but increased frequency of masturbation (Bogaert & Sadava, 2002). As Mikulincer and Shaver (2016) note, this solitary activity of masturbation is consistent with the deactivating strategy of excessive self-reliance, and serves to minimize threats associated with intimacy and closeness. Avoidant individuals also hold attitudes towards sex that make intimacy and closeness less likely; they hold more positive attitudes toward casual sex (Brennan & Shaver, 1995), report greater interest in emotionless sex and uncommitted sexual activities (Gillath & Schachner, 2006), and do not engage in sexual behaviour to enhance intimacy (Schachner & Shaver, 2004). This reluctance to be sexually intimate with partners can place established relationships at risk, and is also likely to interfere with the formation of long-term intimate romantic relationships.

The interpersonal style of avoidant individuals features a reluctance to get close to others, and serves to maintain emotional distance. Those high in attachment avoidance interact with friends less frequently (Gallo & Matthews, 2006) and spend more time alone (Bartholomew & Horowitz, 1991; Shaver et al., 1996). They are also socially inhibited, using less self-disclosure during interactions (Mikulincer & Nachshon, 1991) and having reduced capacity to engage others in conversation that facilitates their disclosure (Bradford, Feeney, & Campbell, 2002). Those high in avoidance display less non-verbal intimacy, affection, closeness, and expressiveness during interactions (Mikulincer & Shaver, 2016). They also use less physical touch, feel uncomfortable with physical touch from others, and report more boredom during interactions compared to secure or anxious individuals (Mikulincer & Shaver, 2016; Tidwell, Reis, & Shaver, 1996). In a behavioural study of attachment-style differences in communication, Guerrero (1996) found that avoidant individuals sat farthest away from partners during interactions, displayed lower receptivity, less gaze, vocal pleasantness, and facial pleasantness, and reduced interest and attentiveness in conversations compared to secure people.

In summary, attachment avoidance is characterized by cognitive, affective, and behavioural processes that undermine intimacy and closeness, and are associated with relational instability, casual sexual encounters, and demonstrations of low romantic interest to prospective partners. Therefore, we have argued that one sub-group of long-term singles may well be characterized by attachment avoidance (Pepping et al., 2018). Next, we consider the mental health outcomes for this sub-group of singles.

## *Mental health implications*

We have argued that the attachment avoidant sub-group of singles will likely display poorer life outcomes and be at risk of poorer mental health (Pepping & MacDonald, 2019). Specifically, although individuals high in attachment avoidance downplay the importance of intimacy, they still desire close relationships (Carvallo & Gabriel, 2006). Indeed, they are even more strongly affected by separation and rejection from close others than their secure counterparts (Feeney & Kirkpatrick, 1996; Fraley, Davis, & Shaver, 1998). This need for intimacy, coupled with the processes that undermine capacity for intimacy and closeness, has been associated with a range of negative life outcomes for avoidant individuals, including loneliness, depression, and reduced life satisfaction (Mikulincer & Shaver, 2016). Further, the characteristic features of attachment avoidance are pervasive and also undermine intimacy in non-romantic relationships (e.g., Mikulincer & Shaver, 2012).

Is it, however, always the case that those who are long-term single due to attachment system deactivation fare worse than their partnered and/or secure counterparts? Avoidant individuals prefer more solitary activities, and it is possible that success in these activities might compensate to some degree for deficits in social connection and intimacy. Indeed, early qualitative research suggests that some people report being long-term single because they are dedicated to career pursuits and work commitments (Forsyth & Johnson, 1995). Interestingly, avoidant individuals can be more successful in careers that are characterized by more self-reliance and autonomy, and may even be more satisfied in this work, compared to their less avoidant counterparts (Ein-Dor, Reizer, Shaver, & Dotan, 2012). Perhaps career success and job satisfaction moderate associations between singlehood and mental health outcomes amongst avoidant individuals.

If career success and job satisfaction do indeed buffer the negative effects of attachment avoidance amongst long-term singles, it seems likely that the protective qualities associated with career success might be attenuated following retirement. A longitudinal study followed workers from pre-retirement to seven years post-retirement and examined the effects of retirement and, in particular, income decline, on physical and mental health (Segel-Karpas, Bamberger, & Bacharach, 2013). Although most individuals coped well following retirement, for those high in attachment avoidance, income decline predicted higher rates of depression, and more psychosomatic complaints and diagnosed illnesses. Thus, avoidant individuals may focus on career pursuits rather than emotional intimacy, in part, to avoid potential vulnerability and disappointment in relationships (see Spielmann et al., 2013), though this strategy may become less effective upon retirement. These findings have important implications for public policy. For instance, the development of post-retirement employment programs, often referred to as bridge employment, may be particularly beneficial for this sub-group upon retirement. Such programs may be an effective method by which avoidant singles, whose career had been a central part of their identity, can continue to meet their needs for accomplishment, recognition, or a sense of meaning and purpose post-retirement (Beehr & Bennett, 2015).

Recent research from our own labs highlights that some people utilize social surrogates, such as non-human objects or fictional characters, to fulfil relational needs and buffer the effects of isolation (Rain, Cilento, MacDonald, & Mar, 2017; see also Derrick, Gabriel, & Hugenberg, 2009). We argued that such strategies may be particularly appealing to those who are insecurely attached, as they involve low risk of rejection and less personal investment (Rain et al., 2017). For instance, individuals high in both attachment anxiety and avoidance more readily engage in narrative transportation, or absorption in a fictional narrative world, such as the world of a fictional character from a television show (Rain et al., 2017). Such absorption might provide an avoidant individual with the experience of emotional closeness with a fictional character, without the risks associated with intimacy in human relationships. It remains unclear whether engagement with fictional narratives and characters actually fulfils an individual's attachment needs. Nonetheless, it seems plausible that engagement with social surrogates, such as narrative transportation, could buffer, or moderate, the negative effects of long-term singlehood amongst insecurely attached individuals to the extent that these social surrogates fulfil an individual's attachment needs. Research is needed to examine whether avoidant long-term singles engage the use of social surrogates, whether use of social surrogates fulfils an individual's need for intimacy, and whether it buffers the effects of social isolation on life satisfaction and well-being.

It is important to consider the potential influence of age and developmental stages when considering mental health outcomes associated with long-term singlehood. Adolescent and early adult relationships are often brief, and many remain single during these early years, which is not associated with poor outcomes (Collins, Welsh, & Furman, 2009). Rather, romantic involvement in adolescence can be associated with poorer outcomes (Olson & Crosnoe, 2017). Therefore, singlehood in early adulthood may be more normative and not associated with attachment insecurity. Consistent with this proposition, Petrowski and colleagues (2015) found that younger single people (aged 18–30) were *more* comfortable with closeness (low avoidance) than their coupled counterparts, whereas older single adults (aged 46–60) were less comfortable with closeness (high avoidance) than their coupled peers. Thus, attachment avoidance may be less predictive of singlehood during adolescence, and in younger individuals, not associated with poor mental health.

Earlier we proposed that some avoidant individuals may adopt strategies to cope with long-term singlehood and isolation more broadly, such as immersion in work or use of social surrogates. However, adopting these strategies might become less effective at alleviating isolation as one ages and requires more social and practical support; this is likely to be especially true for avoidant individuals who are reluctant to seek support in times of need (Vogel & Wei, 2005). Given that social support buffers effects of stressors on overall life satisfaction in older age (e.g., Adams et al., 2016), it seems likely that solitary coping strategies may become less effective as one ages. Interestingly, avoidant attachment predicts lower satisfaction with support received from others among older adults (35–66) but not their younger counterparts (18–34); further, low perceptions of support mediate the effect of avoidant attachment on poor mental health and loneliness in older adulthood (Kafetsios & Sideridis, 2006). Therefore, for avoidant long-term singles, the use of individualistic coping strategies might buffer the effects of isolation on life outcomes in young adulthood, but such strategies likely will become less effective over time. Regarding potential policy implications, programs that offer social and instrumental support in a flexible manner may well be useful here. For instance, Norman (2018) describes a program, run in an independent retirement home in Holland, whereby some residents are students who are able to live in the facility rent-free, in exchange for about 30 hours per month of being a "good neighbour" to the older people living in the facility. The types of activities they provide vary widely, from having conversations at mealtimes, to skill sharing and more practical forms of support, such as teaching older residents to use Skype and email. Such programs may be especially useful for avoidant older adults, as it enables them to determine the type of support and interaction they desire, as well as the level of intimacy with younger residents, ranging from mealtime conversations, to less intimate and more practical forms of support.

## *Anxious attachment and singlehood*

Attachment anxiety is characterized by cognitive, affective, and behavioural processes that undermine success in interpersonal relationships, and may thus prevent the development of stable, satisfying, romantic relationships. Those high in attachment anxiety strongly desire proximity and closeness to romantic partners, but expect that their desire to enhance intimacy will not be reciprocated by relationship partners (Brennan & Shaver, 1995). They are fearful of abandonment and emotional disengagement from partners, and can make demands for reassurance of being loved. They tend to report believing in love at first sight, have frequent experiences of falling in love, and experience love as a form of obsession and desire for merging with the other; however, they also report rarely finding the type of love that meets their expectations (Hazan & Shaver, 1987).

Their strong need for connection, coupled with a view of self as unlovable, leads them to become hypervigilant to threat-related cues (Ein-Dor, Mikulincer, Doron, & Shaver, 2010), and to interpret ambiguous messages in negative ways (Collins & Feeney, 2004). These information processing biases are associated with emotion dysregulation and behavioural patterns that undermine interpersonal success. When the attachment system is activated, anxious individuals experience heightened emotionality and difficulty regulating emotion (Shaver & Mikulincer, 2009). Attachment anxiety is associated with chronic worry about disapproval and rejection, and sensitivity to hurt feelings in relationships (Mikulincer & Shaver, 2016). They tend to also feel overwhelmed by feelings of jealousy, report suspicion of partners, and feel insecure when separated from partners (Mikulincer & Shaver, 2012). As Collins and Feeney (2004) note, this persistent jealousy likely impairs their capacity to be responsive and empathic to the needs of others. Indeed, attachment anxiety is associated with less capacity to be sensitive and responsive to the needs of romantic partners, and predicts compulsive over-caregiving and heightened focus on their own distress when others require support (see Mikulincer & Shaver, 2016).

Individuals high in attachment anxiety experience heightened distress in response to relationship dissolution, and are more likely to perseverate and maintain emotional attachments to previous partners (Davis et al., 2003). Research from our own labs suggests that maintaining intense emotional attachments to previous partners predicts future relationship instability (Spielmann, Joel, MacDonald, & Kogan, 2013). They are also more likely to search for a new partner to reduce distress following break-up (Davis et al., 2003), and this appears to be somewhat effective at reducing their perseveration on ex-partners in the short term (Spielmann, MacDonald, & Wilson, 2009). However, experiences of relationship dissolution reinforce fears of abandonment and rejection for those high in attachment anxiety (Davis et al., 2003).

Those who are high in attachment anxiety are hypervigilant to potential threats in relationships, and tend to be more accurate at inferring a partner's thoughts and emotions in relationship-threatening situations (Simpson et al., 2011). During interactions with potential partners, those who are high in attachment anxiety, consistent with their desire to enhance intimacy, display interest, receptivity, and attentiveness (Guerrero, 1996). Nonetheless, they also engage in behaviours that undermine the success of these interactions (e.g., McClure, Lydon, Baccus, & Baldwin, 2010; McClure & Lydon, 2014). For instance, they tend to present themselves to others in a helpless and self-devaluing way (Mikulincer, 1998), presumably with the goal of eliciting support and enhancing closeness. They display less topical reciprocity when interacting with others, make fewer statements about what the other person has said (Mikulincer & Nachshon, 1991), and are prone to excessive reassurance seeking (Shaver, Schachner, & Mikulincer, 2005). Attachment anxiety is associated with greater romantic jealousy, clinginess, and frustration with relationship partners (Brennan & Shaver, 1995).

In three studies, McClure and Lydon (2014) examined whether attachment anxiety would predict interpersonal failure during interactions, and the behavioural mechanisms underlying this. Those high in attachment anxiety were rated by potential partners as less attractive during a speed-dating session (Study 1) and were rated lower on interpersonal appeal by trained observers (Studies 2 and 3). These effects were mediated by signs of manifest anxiety, verbal disfluencies, interpersonal awkwardness, and social disengagement. In brief, despite strong motivation to connect with others, the cognitive and emotional processes pertaining to fear of abandonment and rejection result in behaviours that impede interpersonal success. These processes are particularly salient when interacting with potential partners as the attachment system is likely to be activated. In summary, attachment anxiety is associated with a range of processes that undermine the quality of close relationships, and we have argued that a second sub-group of long-term singles may be characterized by attachment anxiety (Pepping et al., 2018).

## *Mental health implications*

Those who remain long-term single due to attachment system hyperactivation are likely to be at higher risk of poor mental health. Specifically, those high in attachment anxiety strongly desire close relationships (Hazan & Shaver, 1987; Mikulincer & Shaver, 2016), and are therefore likely to be less satisfied being single, which predicts reduced life satisfaction (Lehmann et al., 2015). Our own research highlights that those who are high in attachment anxiety tend to report more fear of being single, which refers to distress and anxiety about being without a romantic partner (Spielmann, Maxwell et al., 2013). Those who are more fearful of being single are more likely to long for ex-partners (Spielmann, MacDonald, Joel, & Impett, 2015), and are at greater risk of loneliness and depression (Spielmann, Joel et al., 2013). In brief, this sub-group is likely to experience poorer life outcomes, and may experience greater loneliness, compared to those who are single by choice, and compared to their partnered counterparts. Much evidence attests to the negative effects of social isolation and loneliness on indices of mental and physical health (e.g., Holt-Lunstad, Smith, & Layton, 2010; Cacioppo, Hawkley, & Thisted, 2010; Cacioppo, Hughes, Waite, Hawkley, & Thisted, 2006). Nonetheless, there may be factors that affect the association between singlehood and mental health outcomes amongst anxious individuals.

Given that those high in attachment anxiety strongly desire intimacy, some may seek out non-romantic relationships to fulfil attachment needs, and this might buffer the negative effects of singlehood on mental health. For instance, people with broad social ties are less prone to depression (Cruwys et al., 2013), and close friendships can protect against loneliness (Asher & Weeks, 2012). Of particular importance, singles tend to be more socially connected to friends, neighbours, and family members compared to those who are married (Sarkisian & Gerstel, 2016), and thus anxiously attached singles who successfully form long-term relationships with non-romantic partners may not be at risk of poor mental health. It is important to note, however, that attachment anxiety is pervasive and undermines not only romantic relationships, but also non-romantic relationships (e.g., Mikulincer & Shaver, 2012). Thus, the extent to which anxious long-term singles form stable and satisfying long-term friendships, and whether this protects against loneliness, remains unclear.

Regarding public policy implications, involvement in formal organizations might alleviate loneliness and provide anxious long-term singles with some of the social connection they desire. For instance, engagement in volunteer work has well-established benefits to well-being, particularly amongst older adults (e.g., Van Willigen, 2000; Musick & Wilson, 2003) and those who are less socially integrated (Piliavin & Siegl, 2007). Further, social integration (Musick & Wilson, 2003) and feeling valued by others (Piliavin & Siegl, 2007) have each been shown to mediate the effects of volunteering on indices of adjustment. Importantly, the benefits of volunteering are observed amongst both single and married individuals (Morrow-Howell, Hong, & Tang, 2009) suggesting that long-term singles engaged in volunteering may fare just as well as their coupled or single by choice counterparts. Research examining the extent to which social ties and community involvement activities, such as volunteering, moderate the association between long-term singlehood and well-being amongst those high in attachment anxiety would be valuable.

Finally, a large body of evidence reveals that pet ownership can decrease loneliness and increase well-being, particularly for those who may be more socially isolated (e.g., McConnell, Brown, Shoda, Stayton, & Martin, 2011). Importantly, pets are targets for proximity seeking and serve both the secure base and safe haven functions of the attachment system (Zilcha-Mano, Mikulincer, & Shaver, 2011). Pet ownership may thus assist those high in attachment anxiety to cope with loneliness and social isolation, though the benefits of pets tend to be more pronounced amongst securely attached individuals (e.g., Zilcha-Mano, Mikulincer, & Shaver, 2012). Emerging evidence suggests that pet ownership may attenuate loneliness among older adults living alone (Stanley, Conwell, Bowen, & Van Orden, 2014), though there are mixed findings regarding benefits of pet ownership among older adults (Parslow, Jorm, Christensen, Rodgers, & Jacomb, 2005). Again, an individual difference perspective may be clarifying here, and research is needed to investigate whether pet ownership moderates associations between singlehood and life outcomes amongst anxious long-term singles.

## *Secure attachment and singlehood*

We have previously argued that, at least for some, long-term singlehood may not result from attachment insecurity and difficulties in relationships (Pepping et al., 2018; Pepping & MacDonald, 2019). Rather, for some, singlehood may be a personal choice associated with attachment security, with attachment needs being met in other non-romantic relationships. As mentioned earlier, people can form attachments to others outside of romantic relationships (Mikulincer & Shaver, 2016). Thus, some may choose to remain single as their attachment needs are successfully met in other relationships. This possibility has been raised previously (e.g., DePaulo, 2014; Schachner et al., 2008), and qualitative sociological studies suggest at least some individuals choose to remain single and are satisfied with this choice (Band-Winterstein & Manchik-Rimon, 2014; Forsyth & Johnson, 1995).

A qualitative study of 26 long-term single individuals reported two general pathways into singlehood, namely chosen singlehood and constrained singlehood (Timonen & Doyle, 2014). *Chosen singlehood* was characterized by a sense of personal autonomy, self-fulfilment, and satisfaction with single status, whereas *constrained* or involuntary singlehood was characterized by regret and dissatisfaction with one's single status. Recent quantitative research reports similar findings, with satisfaction with single status being associated with greater life satisfaction and less psychological distress compared to those who are less satisfied (Lehmann et al., 2015). Thus, the extent to which singlehood is a choice appears to be critically important when considering mental health and well-being outcomes associated with single status.

What factors influence the choice to remain single? The available research suggests that the reasons vary substantially, and include spiritual and religious reasons, prioritizing career pursuits, and a preference for solitude (e.g., Band-Winterstein & Manchik-Rimon, 2014; Forsyth &

Johnson, 1995; Timonen & Doyle, 2014). We have argued that the specific reason for choosing to remain single may not be overly important (Pepping et al., 2018). Rather, what appears to be critical in determining satisfaction with single status is the extent to which being single reflects a personal choice, as opposed to an involuntary situation one finds themselves in (Forsyth & Johnson, 1995; Lehmann et al., 2015).

In addition, we suggest that the extent to which attachment needs are successfully met in non-romantic relationships is important. People who choose to remain single are still likely to desire some degree of intimacy and closeness, and much evidence attests to the negative effects of social isolation and loneliness (e.g., Holt-Lunstad et al., 2010). Interestingly, research on singlehood from our own labs suggests that having meaningful relationships with non-romantic individuals, such as friends and family members, was the most frequently cited reason for comfort with singlehood (Spielmann, Joel et al., 2013). Thus, the extent to which one has close relationships with others also appears to influence satisfaction with being single, and we suggest that this is a key component of remaining single by choice. The available evidence suggests that the proportion of people for whom singlehood reflects a choice may be reasonably small. Specifically, only 13.2% (Lehmann et al., 2015), and 11% (Forsyth & Johnson, 1995) of singles reported not wishing to be in a relationship or not wanting to marry, respectively.

## *Mental health implications*

When singlehood represents a secure personal choice, as opposed to defensive denial of intimacy needs (as in attachment avoidance), or processes that undermine interpersonal success (as in attachment anxiety), it is likely to be associated with positive psychosocial outcomes. Specifically, individuals who choose to remain single are likely to fare just as well as their (satisfied) partnered counterparts. Consistent with this proposition, Lehmann and colleagues (2015) found that satisfaction with single status was a strong predictor of overall life satisfaction.

Securely attached individuals use the primary attachment strategy of proximity seeking, and they are therefore likely to be motivated to form non-romantic relationships, and may have greater success in these endeavours (Mikulincer & Shaver, 2012). Accordingly, secure individuals who are long-term single may require less assistance in forming and maintaining non-romantic social connections. Broader social ties and fulfilling interpersonal relationships have consistently been associated with increased well-being, less depression, and lower mortality risk (e.g., Cruwys, Haslam, Dingle, Haslam, & Jetten, 2014; Holt-Lunstad et al., 2010). Thus, when singlehood results from a personal choice, rather than difficulties forming and maintaining relationships as in attachment insecurity, those who are long-term single should experience positive mental health outcomes.

## Research challenges, future directions, and lessons learnt

### *Relationship status and mental health outcomes*

As highlighted earlier, attachment security is a positive personal resource in adult romantic relationships, whereas attachment insecurity undermines the quality of relationships (Mikulincer & Shaver, 2016). In our attachment theoretical model of long-term singlehood, we reviewed evidence suggestive of at least three major sub-groups of long-term singles, and outlined how the sub-groups may differentially predict mental health outcomes. An important question that remains unanswered, however, is what differentiates insecure individuals who remain long-term single from those who enter into romantic relationships? Much evidence reveals individuals high in attachment anxiety and avoidance *do* form relationships, albeit relatively less stable and less satisfying ones (Mikulincer & Shaver, 2016). It may be a matter of degree, with those very high in attachment anxiety or avoidance experiencing greater difficulty forming and maintaining romantic relationships. This parallels research on why some dissatisfied couples separate, while others do not. Gottman (1993) argues that what separates those who stay in unhappy relationships from those who do not appears to be the degree of distress and dissatisfaction, and the seriousness of the problems. It seems reasonable that the same may apply to attachment insecurity and long-term singlehood, and future research should address this question.

Similarly, it remains unclear what factors may differentiate securely attached individuals who remain long-term single from those who enter into relationships. We have argued that some securely attached individuals may choose to remain single, and have their attachment needs met in relationships outside of romantic pair-bonds. Perhaps there are individual difference characteristics that have influence on this decision. One such factor may be an unrestricted sociosexual orientation, referring to comfort with casual sexual encounters in the absence of love and long-term commitment (Simpson & Gangestad, 1992). It seems possible that individuals with a secure attachment style who also prefer casual sexual encounters rather than long-term committed relationships may choose to remain single, and have their sexual needs met in relationships other than romantic pair-bonds. Research is needed to test the interaction between attachment security and sociosexual orientation and its association with the decision to remain long-term single.

It is necessary to consider the impact of context on singlehood, particularly in relation to sub-groups of singles. There have been major social changes in recent years that have likely impacted upon the rise in singlehood. For instance, there are now technologies to assist with reproduction, including surrogate mothers and in vitro fertilization, meaning those who do not wish to be in a romantic relationship (i.e., singlehood as a choice) are able to have children in the absence of a relationship. Similarly, the economic need for women to enter into committed relationships has decreased with the increasing education and employment opportunities for women (Carr, 2002). At the same time, the increasing acceptability of casual sex (Garcia, Reiber, Massey, & Merriwether, 2012) may enable those who wish to have sexual relationships in the absence of romantic pair-bonds to do so more readily. In brief, there is less of a financial, sexual, and reproductive imperative to form long-term committed relationships, which likely explains at least some of the increase in singlehood, particularly amongst those for whom singlehood reflects a personal choice.

There are additional societal changes that likely interfere with the development of romantic relationships. People in the Western world are increasingly living alone and are less connected to family units and community (Orum, Johnstone, & Riger, 1999). Adults in Western societies are becoming less empathic (Konrath, O'Brien, & Hsing, 2011) and display less need for social approval from others (Twenge & Im, 2007). It appears that the Western world is becoming increasingly individualistic, and this is supported by evidence of an increase in individualistic words (e.g., "independence" and "self-reliance") and phrases (e.g., "all about me" and "I am special") in American literature between 1960 and 2008 (Twenge, Campbell, & Gentile, 2012). The two dimensions of attachment insecurity are also associated with less empathic concern for others, greater self-focus, and higher narcissism (Mikulincer & Shaver, 2016). It seems likely that these societal changes may be particularly pronounced and problematic amongst those with a predisposition to such characteristics (i.e., high attachment anxiety and avoidance). In brief, not only has there been a large increase in attachment insecurity in recent years (Konrath, Chopik, Hsing, & O'Brien, 2014), attachment insecurity likely interacts with widespread social changes, with those predisposed to difficulties in relationships being most at risk of isolation in an increasingly individualistic culture.

### *Intervention*

We believe psychology has much to offer regarding intervention for those who wish to enter into romantic relationships, but struggle to do so. There are well-established, evidence-based, couple relationship education programs (Halford & Bodenmann, 2013) and two empirically supported couple therapy approaches (Snyder & Halford, 2012) designed to help *couples* develop relationship skills and knowledge, and have more satisfying relationships. Early psychological research trialled "practice dating" behavioural interventions for anxious, socially inhibited college students (e.g., Christensen & Arkowitz, 1974; Christensen, Arkowitz, & Anderson, 1975). Although these studies generally reported beneficial effects, participants were young college students rather than long-term singles, and effects were examined only at two-week and three-month follow-ups.

Evidence-based relationship education could be beneficial for long-term singles who desire a relationship. For instance, relationship education programs promote realistic relationship expectations, teach relationship skills such as communication and conflict resolution, and enhance relationship self-regulation, whereby individuals reflect on aspects of their own behaviour they wish to change to enhance their relationship (Halford & Bodenmann, 2013). It is plausible that an educative intervention to teach relationship knowledge and skills could benefit long-term singles who desire a relationship. We are not aware of any empirically validated intervention that assists those wishing to enter a romantic relationship resolve the difficulties that prevent them from doing so; this probably reflects the scarce psychological research dedicated to understanding singlehood, which is necessary for intervention development.

## Conclusions

In this chapter, we have outlined how humans have a fundamental need for social relationships, and the quality of these relationships is a strong predictor of mental health and well-being. Our own work has focused on understanding romantic relationships and singlehood from an attachment perspective. The challenge for researchers now is to better understand the mental health implications of singlehood, with particular focus on variability within this heterogeneous group. Further, the ways in which individual differences in attachment might interact with broad societal changes in the Western world, and the mental health implications of these interactions, is a topic in need of further research. Finally, there is a need to develop programs that assist those who remain long-term single to fulfil their attachment needs in other ways. Similarly, there is a great need for research to develop and evaluate interventions that help people form and maintain satisfying relationships over time.

## References

Adamczyk, K., & Bookwala, J. (2013). Adult attachment and single vs. partnered relationship status in Polish university students. *Psychological Topics*, *22*(3), 481–500.

Adams, T. R., Rabin, L. A., Da Silva, V. G., Katz, M. J., Fogel, J., & Lipton, R. B. (2016). Social support buffers the impact of depressive symptoms on life satisfaction in old age. *Clinical Gerontologist*, *39*(2), 139–157.

Asher, S. R., & Weeks, M. S. (2012). Social relationships, academic engagement, and well-being in college: Findings from the Duke social relationships project. Retrieved from https://sites.duke.edu/dsrp/files/2011/10/DSRP-Report-FINALrev1.pdf

Australian Institute of Family Studies. (2019). Marriage in Australia source data. Retrieved from https://aifs.gov.au/facts-and-figures/marriage-australia/marriage-australia-source-data

Band-Winterstein, T., & Manchik-Rimon, C. (2014). The experience of being an old never-married single: A life course perspective. *The International Journal of Aging and Human Development*, *78*(4), 379–401.

Bartholomew, K., & Horowitz, L. M. (1991). Attachment styles among young adults: A test of a four-category model. *Journal of Personality and Social Psychology*, *61*(2), 226–244.

Baumeister, R. F., & Leary, M. R. (1995). The need to belong: Desire for interpersonal attachments as a fundamental human motivation. *Psychological Bulletin*, *117*(3), 497–529.

Beehr, T. A., & Bennett, M. M. (2015). Working after retirement: Features of bridge employment and research directions. *Work, Aging and Retirement*, *1*(1), 112–128.

Bogaert, A. F., & Sadava, S. (2002). Adult attachment and sexual behavior. *Personal Relationships*, *9*(2), 191–204.

Bowlby, J. (1969). *Attachment and loss, Vol. 1: Attachment*. New York, NY: Basic Books.

Bowlby, J. (1973). *Attachment and loss, Vol. 2: Separation, anxiety and anger*. London: Hogarth Press.

Bowlby, J. (1980). *Attachment and loss, Vol. 3: Sadness and depression – attachment and loss*. London: Hogarth Press

Bradford, S. A., Feeney, J. A., & Campbell, L. (2002). Links between attachment orientations and dispositional and diary – based measures of disclosure in dating couples: A study of actor and partner effects. *Personal Relationships*, *9*(4), 491–506.

Brennan, K. A., & Shaver, P. R. (1995). Dimensions of adult attachment, affect regulation, and romantic relationship functioning. *Personality and Social Psychology Bulletin*, *21*(3), 267–283.

Cacioppo, J. T., Hawkley, L. C., & Thisted, R. A. (2010). Perceived social isolation makes me sad: 5-Year cross-lagged analyses of loneliness and depressive symptomatology in the Chicago health, aging, and social relations study. *Psychology and Aging*, *25*(2), 453–463.

Cacioppo, J. T., Hughes, M. E., Waite, L. J., Hawkley, L. C., & Thisted, R. A. (2006). Loneliness as a specific risk factor for depressive symptoms: Cross-sectional and longitudinal analyses. *Psychology and Aging*, *21*(1), 140–151.

Carr, D. (2002). The psychological consequences of work-family trade-offs for three cohorts of men and women. *Social Psychology Quarterly*, 103–124.

Carvallo, M., & Gabriel, S. (2006). No man is an island: The need to belong and dismissing avoidant attachment style. *Personality and Social Psychology Bulletin*, *32*(5), 697–709.

Cassidy, J., & Shaver, P. R. (2016). *Adult attachment: Theory, research, and clinical applications*. New York, NY: Guilford Press.

Christensen, A., & Arkowitz, H. (1974). Preliminary report on practice dating and feedback as treatment for college dating problems. *Journal of Counseling Psychology*, *21*(2), 92–95.

Christensen, A., Arkowitz, H., & Anderson, J. (1975). Practice dating as treatment for college dating inhibitions. *Behaviour Research and Therapy*, *13*(4), 321–331.

Collins, N. L., & Feeney, B. C. (2004). Working models of attachment shape perceptions of social support: Evidence from experimental and observational studies. *Journal of Personality and Social Psychology*, *87*(3), 363–383.

Collins, W. A., Welsh, D. P., & Furman, W. (2009). Adolescent romantic relationships. *Annual Review of Psychology*, *60*, 631–652.

Cruwys, T., Dingle, G. A., Haslam, C., Haslam, S. A., Jetten, J., & Morton, T. A. (2013). Social group memberships protect against future depression, alleviate depression symptoms and prevent depression relapse. *Social Science & Medicine*, *98*, 179–186.

Cruwys, T., Haslam, S. A., Dingle, G. A., Haslam, C., & Jetten, J. (2014). Depression and social identity: An integrative review. *Personality and Social Psychology Review*, *18*, 215–238.

Davis, D., Shaver, P. R., & Vernon, M. L. (2003). Physical, emotional, and behavioral reactions to breaking up: The roles of gender, age, emotional involvement, and attachment style. *Personality and Social Psychology Bulletin, 29*(7), 871–884.

DePaulo, B. (2014). A singles studies perspective on mount marriage. *Psychological Inquiry, 25*, 64–68. doi:10.1080/1047840X.2014.878173

DePaulo, B. M., & Morris, W. L. (2005). Singles in society and in science. *Psychological Inquiry, 16*(2–3), 57–83.

Derrick, J. L., Gabriel, S., & Hugenberg, K. (2009). Social surrogacy: How favored television programs provide the experience of belonging. *Journal of Experimental Social Psychology, 45*(2), 352–362.

Diener, E., Suh, E. M., Lucas, R. E., & Smith, H. L. (1999). Subjective well-being: Three decades of progress. *Psychological Bulletin, 125*(2), 276–302.

Ein-Dor, T., Mikulincer, M., Doron, G., & Shaver, P. R. (2010). The attachment paradox: How can so many of us (the insecure ones) have no adaptive advantages? *Perspectives on Psychological Science, 5*(2), 123–141.

Ein-Dor, T., Reizer, A., Shaver, P. R., & Dotan, E. (2012). Standoffish perhaps, but successful as well: Evidence that avoidant attachment can be beneficial in professional tennis and computer science. *Journal of Personality, 80*(3), 749–768.

Feeney, B. C., & Kirkpatrick, L. A. (1996). Effects of adult attachment and presence of romantic partners on physiological responses to stress. *Journal of Personality and Social Psychology, 70*(2), 255–270.

Fisher, H. E., Aron, A., & Brown, L. L. (2006). Romantic love: A mammalian brain system for mate choice. *Philosophical Transactions of the Royal Society B: Biological Sciences, 361*(1476), 2173–2186.

Fletcher, G. J., Simpson, J. A., Campbell, L., & Overall, N. C. (2015). Pair-bonding, romantic love, and evolution: The curious case of homo sapiens. *Perspectives on Psychological Science, 10*(1), 20–36.

Forsyth, C. J., & Johnson, E. L. (1995). A sociological view of the never married. *International Journal of Sociology of the Family*, 91–104.

Fraley, R. C., Davis, K. E., & Shaver, P. R. (1998). Dismissing-avoidance and the defensive organization of emotion, cognition, and behavior. In J. A. Simpson & W. S. Rholes (Eds.), *Attachment theory and close relationships* (pp. 249–279). New York, NY: Guilford Press.

Fraley, R. C., Waller, N. G., & Brennan, K. A. (2000). An item-response theory analysis of self-report measures of attachment. *Journal of Personality and Social Psychology, 78*(2), 350–365.

Gallo, L. C., & Matthews, K. A. (2006). Adolescents' attachment orientation influences ambulatory blood pressure responses to everyday social interactions. *Psychosomatic Medicine, 68*(2), 253–261.

Garcia, J. R., Reiber, C., Massey, S. G., & Merriwether, A. M. (2012). Sexual hookup culture: A review. *Review of General Psychology, 16*(2), 161–176.

Gillath, O., & Schachner, D. A. (2006). How do sexuality and attachment interrelate? Goals, motives and strategies. In M. Mikulincer & G. Goodman

(Eds.), *Dynamics of romantic love: Attachment, caregiving, and sex* (pp. 337–355). New York, NY: Guilford Press.

Gottman, J. M. (1993). *What predicts divorce? The relationship between marital processes and marital outcomes*. New York, NY: Psychology Press.

Guerrero, L. K. (1996). Attachment-style differences in intimacy and involvement: A test of the four-category model. *Communications Monographs, 63*(4), 269–292.

Halford, W. K., & Bodenmann, G. (2013). Effects of relationship education on maintenance of couple relationship satisfaction. *Clinical Psychology Review, 33*(4), 512–525.

Hazan, C., & Shaver, P. (1987). Romantic love conceptualized as an attachment process. *Journal of Personality and Social Psychology, 52*(3), 511–524.

Holmes, J. (2001). *The search for the secure base: Attachment theory and psychotherapy*. Hove: Brunner-Routledge.

Holt-Lunstad, J., Smith, T. B., & Layton, J. B. (2010). Social relationships and mortality risk: A meta-analytic review. *PLoS Medicine*, 7(7), 859.

Kafetsios, K., & Sideridis, G. D. (2006). Attachment, social support and well-being in young and older adults. *Journal of Health Psychology, 11*(6), 863–875.

Keith, P. M. (1980). Two models of singleness: Managing an atypical marital status. *International Journal of Sociology of the Family*, 301–310.

Kirkpatrick, L. A., & Hazan, C. (1994). Attachment style and close relationships: A four year prospective study. *Personal Relationships, 1*(2), 123–142.

Konrath, S. H., Chopik, W. J., Hsing, C. K., & O'Brien, E. (2014). Changes in adult attachment styles in American college students over time a meta-analysis. *Personality and Social Psychology Review, 18*(4), 326–348.

Konrath, S. H., O'Brien, E. H., & Hsing, C. (2011). Changes in dispositional empathy in American college students over time: A meta-analysis. *Personality and Social Psychology Review, 15*(2), 180–198.

Kurdek, L. A. (1991). The relations between reported well-being and divorce history, availability of a proximate adult, and gender. *Journal of Marriage and the Family*, 71–78.

Lehmann, V., Tuinman, M. A., Braeken, J., Vingerhoets, A. J., Sanderman, R., & Hagedoorn, M. (2015). Satisfaction with relationship status: Development of a new scale and the role in predicting well-being. *Journal of Happiness Studies, 16*(1), 169–184.

Lucas, R. E., & Dyrenforth, P. S. (2005). The myth of marital bliss? *Psychological Inquiry*, 111–115.

Main, M. (1990). Cross-cultural studies of attachment organization: Recent studies, changing methodologies, and the concept of conditional strategies. *Human Development, 33*(1), 48–61.

McClure, M. J., & Lydon, J. E. (2014). Anxiety doesn't become you: How attachment anxiety compromises relational opportunities. *Journal of Personality and Social Psychology, 106*(1), 89–111.

McClure, M. J., Lydon, J. E., Baccus, J. R., & Baldwin, M. W. (2010). A signal detection analysis of chronic attachment anxiety at speed dating: Being unpopular is only the first part of the problem. *Personality and Social Psychology Bulletin*, *36*, 1024–1026.

McConnell, A. R., Brown, C. M., Shoda, T. M., Stayton, L. E., & Martin, C. E. (2011). Friends with benefits: On the positive consequences of pet ownership. *Journal of Personality and Social Psychology*, *101*(6), 1239–1252.

Mikulincer, M. (1998). Attachment working models and the sense of trust: An exploration of interaction goals and affect regulation. *Journal of Personality and Social* Psychology, *74*, 1209–1224.

Mikulincer, M., & Nachshon, O. (1991). Attachment styles and patterns of self-disclosure. *Journal of Personality and Social Psychology*, *61*(2), 321–331.

Mikulincer, M., & Shaver, P. R. (2007). *Attachment in adulthood: Structure, dynamics, and change*. New York, NY: Guilford Press.

Mikulincer, M., & Shaver, P. R. (2012). Adult attachment orientations and relationship processes. *Journal of Family Theory & Review*, *4*(4), 259–274.

Mikulincer, M., & Shaver, P. R. (2016). *Attachment in adulthood: Structure, dynamics, and change* (2nd ed.). New York, NY: Guilford Press.

Morrow-Howell, N., Hong, S. I., & Tang, F. (2009). Who benefits from volunteering? Variations in perceived benefits. *The Gerontologist*, *49*(1), 91–102.

Musick, M. A., & Wilson, J. (2003). Volunteering and depression: The role of psychological and social resources in different age groups. *Social Science & Medicine*, *56*(2), 259–269.

Norman, C. (2018). Preventing loneliness in older patients. *British Journal of Community Nursing*, *23*(7), 323–325.

Office for National Statistics. (2019). Marriages in England and Wales: 2016. Retrieved from www.ons.gov.uk/peoplepopulationandcommunity/birthsdeathsandmarriages/marriagecohabitationandcivilpartnerships/bulletins/marriagesinenglandandwalesprovisional/2016

Olson, J. S., & Crosnoe, R. (2017). Are you still bringing me down? Romantic involvement and depressive symptoms from adolescence to young adulthood. *Journal of Health and Social Behavior*, *58*(1), 102–115.

Orum, A. M., Johnstone, J. W. C., & Riger, S. (1999). *Changing societies: Essential sociology for our times*. Lanham, MD: Rowman & Littlefield.

Parslow, R. A., Jorm, A. F., Christensen, H., Rodgers, B., & Jacomb, P. (2005). Pet ownership and health in older adults: Findings from a survey of 2,551 community-based Australians aged 60–64. *Gerontology*, *51*(1), 40–47.

Pepping, C. A., & MacDonald, G. (2019). Adult attachment and long-term singlehood. *Current Opinion in Psychology*, *25*, 105–109.

Pepping, C. A., MacDonald, G., & Davis, P. J. (2018). Toward a psychology of singlehood: An attachment-theory perspective on long-term singlehood. *Current Directions in Psychological Science*, *27*(5), 324–331.

Petrowski, K., Schurig, S., Schmutzer, G., Brahler, E., & Stobel-Richter, Y. (2015). Is it attachment style or socio-demography: Singlehood in a representative sample. *Frontiers in Psychology*, *6*, 1738.

Piliavin, J. A., & Siegl, E. (2007). Health benefits of volunteering in the Wisconsin longitudinal study. *Journal of Health and Social Behavior*, *48*(4), 450–464.

Quirk, K., Owen, J., Shuck, B., Fincham, F. D., Knopp, K., & Rhoades, G. (2015). Breaking bad: Commitment uncertainty, alternative monitoring, and relationship termination in young adults. *Journal of Couple & Relationship Therapy*, 1–14.

Rain, M., Cilento, E., MacDonald, G., & Mar, R. A. (2017). Adult attachment and transportation into narrative worlds. *Personal Relationships*, *24*(1), 49–74.

Ringstad, S., & Pepping, C. A. (2016). Attachment and long term singlehood. Poster presented at the World Congress of Behavioural and Cognitive Therapies, Melbourne.

Robles, T. F., Slatcher, R. B., Trombello, J. M., & McGinn, M. M. (2014). Marital quality and health: A meta-analytic review. *Psychological Bulletin*, *140*(1), 140–187.

Sarkisian, N., & Gerstel, N. (2016). Does singlehood isolate or integrate? Examining the link between marital status and ties to kin, friends, and neighbors. *Journal of Social and Personal Relationships*, *33*(3), 361–384.

Sbarra, D. A., Hasselmo, K., & Bourassa, K. J. (2015). Divorce and health: Beyond individual differences. *Current Directions in Psychological Science*, *24*(2), 109–113.

Schachner, D. A., & Shaver, P. R. (2004). Attachment dimensions and sexual motives. *Personal Relationships*, *11*(2), 179–195.

Schachner, D. A., Shaver, P. R., & Gillath, O. (2008). Attachment style and long-term singlehood. *Personal Relationships*, *15*(4), 479–491.

Segel-Karpas, D., Bamberger, P. A., & Bacharach, S. B. (2013). Income decline and retiree well-being: The moderating role of attachment. *Psychology and Aging*, *28*(4), 1098–1107.

Shaver, P. R., & Mikulincer, M. (2009). Adult attachment strategies and the regulation of emotion. In J. J. Gross (Ed.), *Handbook of emotion regulation* (pp. 446–465). New York, NY: Guilford Press.

Shaver, P. R., Papalia, D., Clark, C. L., Koski, L. R., Tidwell, M. C., & Nalbone, D. (1996). Androgyny and attachment security: Two related models of optimal personality. *Personality and Social Psychology Bulletin*, *22*(6), 582–597.

Shaver, P. R., Schachner, D. A., & Mikulincer, M. (2005). Attachment style, excessive reassurance seeking, relationship processes, and depression. *Personality and Social Psychology Bulletin*, *31*(3), 343–359.

Simpson, J. A., & Gangestad, S. W. (1992). Sociosexuality and romantic partner choice. *Journal of Personality*, *60*(1), 31–51.

Simpson, J. A., Kim, J. S., Fillo, J., Ickes, W., Rholes, W. S., Oriña, M. M., & Winterheld, H. A. (2011). Attachment and the management of empathic accuracy in relationship-threatening situations. *Personality and Social Psychology Bulletin*, *37*(2), 242–254.

Snyder, D. K., & Halford, W. K. (2012). Evidence-based couple therapy: Current status and future directions. *Journal of Family Therapy*, *34*(3), 229–249.

Spielmann, S. S., Joel, S., MacDonald, G., & Kogan, A. (2013). Ex appeal current relationship quality and emotional attachment to ex-partners. *Social Psychological and Personality Science*, *4*(2), 175–180.

Spielmann, S. S., MacDonald, G., Joel, S., & Impett, E. A. (2015). Longing for ex-partners out of fear of being single. *Journal of Personality, 84*(6), 799–808.

Spielmann, S. S., MacDonald, G., Maxwell, J. A., Joel, S., Peragine, D., Muise, A., & Impett, E.A. (2013). Settling for less out of fear of being single. *Journal of Personality and Social Psychology, 105*(6), 1049–1073.

Spielmann, S. S., MacDonald, G., & Wilson, A. E. (2009). On the rebound: Focusing on someone new helps anxiously attached individuals let go of ex-partners. *Personality and Social Psychology Bulletin, 35*(10), 1382–1394.

Spielmann, S. S., Maxwell, J. A., MacDonald, G., & Baratta, P. L. (2013). Don't get your hopes up avoidantly attached individuals perceive lower social reward when there is potential for intimacy. *Personality and Social Psychology Bulletin, 39*(2), 219–236.

Stanley, I. H., Conwell, Y., Bowen, C., & Van Orden, K.A. (2014). Pet ownership may attenuate loneliness among older adult primary care patients who live alone. *Aging & Mental Health, 18*(3), 394–399.

Statistics Canada. (2015). Marital status: Overview, 2011. Retrieved from https://www150.statcan.gc.ca/n1/pub/91-209-x/2013001/article/11788-eng.htm

Stein, P. J. (1978). The lifestyles and life chances of the never-married. *Marriage & Family Review, 1*(4), 1–11.

Timonen, V., & Doyle, M. (2014). Life-long singlehood: Intersections of the past and the present. *Ageing and Society, 34*(10), 1749–1770.

Twenge, J. M., Campbell, W. K., & Gentile, B. (2012). Increases in individualistic words and phrases in American books, 1960–2008. *PloS One*, 7(7), e40181.

Twenge, J. M., & Im, C. (2007). Changes in the need for social approval, 1958–2001. *Journal of Research in Personality, 41*(1), 171–189.

U.S. Census Bureau. (1970). Marital status of the population by sex, race, and Hispanic origin. Retrieved from www.allcountries.org/uscensus/53_marital_status_of_the_population_by.html

U.S. Census Bureau. (2011). Statistical abstract: Table 56: Marital status of the population by sex, race, and Hispanic origin: 1990 to 2010. Retrieved from ftp://ftp.census.gov/library/publications/2011/compendia/statab/131ed/tables/12s0056.pdf

U.S. Census Bureau. (2017). Table AD-3: Living arrangements of adults 18 and over, 1967 to present. Retrieved from https://www2.census.gov/programs-surveys/demo/tables/families/time-series/adults/ad3.xlsx

Van Willigen, M. (2000). Differential benefits of volunteering across the life course. *The Journals of Gerontology Series B, 55*(5), S308–S318.

Vogel, D. L., & Wei, M. (2005). Adult attachment and help-seeking intent: The mediating roles of psychological distress and perceived social support. *Journal of Counseling Psychology, 52*(3), 347–357.

Whisman, M. A. (2007). Marital distress and DSM-IV psychiatric disorders in a population-based national survey. *Journal of Abnormal Psychology, 116*(3), 638–643.

Zilcha-Mano, S., Mikulincer, M., & Shaver, P. R. (2011). An attachment perspective on human – pet relationships: Conceptualization and assessment of pet attachment orientations. *Journal of Research in Personality*, *45*(4), 345–357.

Zilcha-Mano, S., Mikulincer, M., & Shaver, P. R. (2012). Pets as safe havens and secure bases: The moderating role of pet attachment orientations. *Journal of Research in Personality*, *46*(5), 571–580.

# 3

# PARENTING, FAMILY ENVIRONMENTS, AND MENTAL HEALTH AND ILLNESS

*James N. Kirby and Cassandra L. Tellegen*

## The context of the research: how parenting creates nurturing family environments

Consistently, parenting researchers have found that coercive, dismissive, and psychological controlling parenting practices (e.g., authoritarian using punitive practices) lead to poorer child outcomes, compared to children who receive positive parenting practices (e.g., warm, responsive; Kaminski, Valle, Filence, & Boyle, 2008; Sanders, Kirby, Tellegen, & Day, 2014). What is surprising, given this knowledge, is that today smacking and corporal punishment – use of an object, such as a paddle (an authoritarian and punitive parenting practice) – are still well-used and accepted parenting practices (D'Souza, Russell, Wood, Signal, & Elder, 2016; Klevens & Whitaker, 2007; Regalado, Sareen, Inkelas, Wissow, & Halfon, 2004). For example, in a recent study of New Zealand parents (D'Souza et al., 2016), researchers found that although smacking and corporal punishment had declined from 89% in 1981, it still had a 40% approval by parents in 2013. This view is echoed in other Western countries such as the United States of America (USA), where 74% report hitting their children (Jackson et al., 1999), and 47% reported hitting very young children (Regalado et al., 2004).

The original Adverse Childhood Experiences (ACEs) study (Felitti et al., 1998) sheds further light on the significance of the problems in home environments. ACEs include three categories: abuse (emotional, physical, sexual), household challenges (mother treated violently, household substance abuse, household mental illness, parental separation or divorce, incarcerated household member), and neglect (emotional and physical). The results from this study that included over 9,508 participants from Kaiser Permanente's San Diego Health Appraisal Clinic in the US found that 64% had at least one ACE as a child. Individuals who had experienced four or more ACEs had a 12-fold increased health risk for alcoholism, drug abuse, depression, and suicide attempts. The study concluded that there was a strong relationship between the number of ACEs experienced during childhood and multiple risk factors of several leading causes of death in adults. Importantly, children raised in hostile family environments are at risk for developing life-long fears of positive emotions and compassion (Matos, Duarte, & Pinto-Gouveia, 2017) and an underdeveloped attachment system (Gilbert, McEwan, Matos, & Rivis, 2010). Conversely, children raised in family environments characterized by warm-rewarding parenting will moderate the genetic contribution to callus-unemotional traits in childhood (Henri et al., 2018).

These results illustrate three key points: 1) that many children today are being raised in '*toxic*' environments, ones which are characterized by threat and not by compassion (Felitti et al., 1998; WHO, 2014); 2) toxic environments have significant impacts on brain-body development and can lead to long-term fears of affiliation and compassion (Biglan, Flay, Embry, & Sandler, 2012; Gilbert et al., 2010); and 3) the need for parents to have access to evidence-based parenting programs to improve parenting practices and childhood outcomes. Yet, the response to childhood distress appears to be somewhat underwhelming, with few governments around the world adopting policies to offer evidence-based parenting programs to help parents raise their children and reduce the prevalence of child maltreatment (Prinz, Sanders, Shapiro, Whitaker, & Lutzker, 2009; Sanders & Kirby, 2014). Importantly, parenting style is modifiable, and over the last 30 years, various parenting programs have been developed to target parental factors of skills and competency to improve outcomes for children (Sanders & Kirby, 2014; Kirby, 2016). Therefore, there is a great need for our communities to invest in helping parents raise their children in a family context that fosters compassion and strengthens a prosocial phenotype, which in turn will benefit childhood physical health, as well as mental and social well-being, and society as a whole.

## *Compassion focused parenting*

One of the most important parenting provisions, to create a safe and supportive environment for children, is to be sensitive to the child's needs and distress and respond appropriately. Indeed, in early childhood the parent is typically the only source of need fulfilment and emotion and distress regulation, as children are vulnerable and lack the required competencies to meet those needs (Seigel & Bryson, 2011; Swain & Ho, 2016). Hence in many ways the various motives and competencies that underpin compassion are crucial to the provision of safe, predictable, and secure environments for children.

Compassion can be defined as "a sensitivity to the suffering in self and others, with a commitment to try and alleviate or prevent it" (Gilbert, 2014). Note that prevention of suffering is important to compassionate motivation. This is especially important for childhood because a parent who is not empathetically sensitive to the needs of their child may cause a lot of suffering. For example, there can be potential neurological damage to the developing brain of babies who are left to cry alone regularly (Bugental, Martorell, & Barraza, 2003; Schore, 1997), and at an extreme, unfed children tend to starve (an all too common occurrence in developing countries where access to food is scarce; Maternal and Child Nutrition Study Group, 2013), both examples of parental neglect.

Compassion involves two key aspects: 1) having a signal detection to suffering (i.e., sensitivity and awareness), and 2) having a signal responsiveness to suffering (i.e., taking some kind of action to alleviate and prevent suffering). Thus, compassion will involve a number of important competencies, such as how to *pay attention*; being emotionally moved by distress calls – that is *sympathy* (rather than being disinterested or irritated by it); having *empathy*, for example knowing that a certain type of crying might mean wanting to eat, versus feeling pain, distress, or tiredness. In addition, as the child develops, knowing when to remove him/her from all anxiety, in contrast to helping the child stay with and cope with that anxiety (e.g., going to school). Thus, parents have to be able to *tolerate distress* and be *non-judgemental* – that is, non-condemning and non-critical (Gilbert, 2014; Seigel & Bryson, 2011). The second component of compassion requires action and skills, and providing parents with specific evidence-based parenting training can be one effective way to help in the social, emotional, and behavioural development of children (Kirby, 2016). Compassion includes three directions: giving compassion to others (e.g., friend, family member), being open and responding to receiving compassion from others, and self-compassion (Gilbert, 2014).

*Compassion focused parenting* is taking a compassion focused therapy (CFT) approach to understanding parenting motivations and behaviours. CFT, developed by Paul Gilbert over the last 20 years (see Gilbert, 2014 for review), is an integrative, evolutionary, contextual, and biopsychosocial approach to understanding the nature of mind and body. CFT focuses on two psychologies of compassion. The first psychology is a motivation to engage with suffering, and the second psychology is focused on action, specifically acting to help alleviate and prevent suffering. CFT is an approach to therapy that emphasizes how the evolved brain was not developed 'perfectly' and rather has a host of complexities and 'trade-offs' that can cause suffering (e.g., shame, criticism, anxiety, depression). The emphasis of CFT is on the *process* of how therapy is delivered, focusing on the various fears, blocks, and resistances people have to compassion, and utilizing physiological processes to help individuals embody change (e.g., body posture, vocal tone, heart rate variability). To date, CFT has been examined in a number of trials, and a systematic review was conducted in 2014 that included 14 evaluation studies (Leaviss & Uttley, 2015). The review concluded that CFT shows promise as an intervention for mood disorders, particularly for those high in self-criticism.

Notably, compassion focused parenting does not simply mean 'being nice' to your children; indeed, a compassion focused parent will, for example, prevent a child from overeating or staying up too late despite protests from the child (this can take some courage and distress tolerance). Indeed, compassion still requires boundaries and consequences; however, these are not enforced in punitive or shaming ways. Having family ground rules is important in creating safety and predictability so parents and children are aware of what to do and what is generally expected. Indeed, there are many times when parenting your child or children is not easy, and the parent can have high levels of self-doubt, stress, and guilt as to what to do in their role as caregiver (Haslam, Patrick, & Kirby, 2015; Kirby, 2016). Thus, compassion focused parenting does require a number of competencies that parents range in their ability to perform (for example distress tolerance). Therefore, in order to best help our children, we must help our parents, and provide them with the skills, knowledge, and confidence of a style of parenting that is compassion focused, as this will help promote well-being in children and parents, whilst preventing and alleviating suffering.

## *The caring system motive and parenting*

Fogel, Melson, and Mistry (1986) provide an influential framework to caring-nurturance and parental investment, which helps facilitate the attachment system. This includes five important capacities: a) an *awareness* of the need to be nurturing; b) a *motivation* to nurture; c) an *understanding* of what is needed to be nurturing; d) having the capacity to *express* nurturing feelings, and e) having *feedback* systems, that is, having the ability to change behaviour depending on whether it has been successful or not (using the previous example of the newborn infant crying, if soothing through touch or voice does not work the parent may need to feed the infant as he/she could have been hungry). This approach to caring and nurturing helps create the attachment system for the child (Bowlby, 1969; Mikulincer & Shaver, 2016). There are three key components to attachment: *proximity seeking* – that is the child's desire to have closeness to an attachment figure (typically mum or dad); *secure base* – the child having a source of security and guidance to go out and explore and develop confidence; and *safe haven* – the child having a source of comfort when distressed to help facilitate emotion regulation (Bowlby, 1969; Mikulincer & Shaver, 2016). The attachment system is critical to mammalian evolution, and particularly for humans, as affiliative emotions and relating to others (e.g., parent, family, friends, others) are potentially the most significant in terms of affect regulation (Gilbert, 2014). Affiliative connection can include touch, facial expression, and voice tone, among a number of other factors (Goetz, Keltner, & Simon-Thomas, 2010; Porges, 2007).

## *Affect regulation in compassion focused parenting*

A key component of compassion focused parenting is understanding emotion systems and affect regulation. Gilbert (2009) proposed that emotion regulation occurs through three systems: threat (e.g., self-protection, safety seeking), drive (e.g., achievement, incentive-focused, status), and soothe (e.g., non-wanting, safeness, interpersonal connection) (see Figure 3.1). One of the aims of CFT is to enhance insight into how individuals automatically respond to threat in defensive ways, which can have negative unintended consequences, such as maladaptive

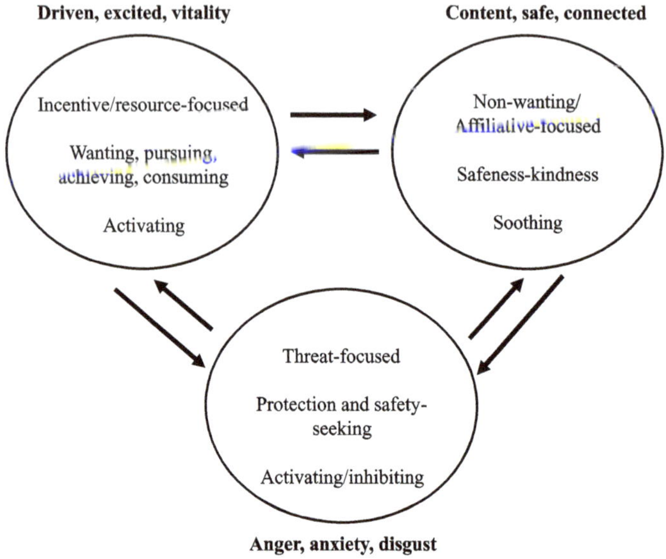


**FIGURE 3.1** The interaction between the three major emotion-regulation systems (from Gilbert, *The Compassionate Mind* (2009), reprinted with permission from Constable & Robinson Ltd)

self-criticism (Carona, Rijo, Ssalvador, Castilho, & Gilbert, 2017). At a deeper level, cognitive processes such as rumination, negativity bias, and self-critical monitoring may reflect evolutionary responses to threat employed by the human brain (Matos et al., 2017). By developing awareness of the tricky interplay between old-brain emotions and new brain-capacities, a context for self-compassion can therefore be created (Gilbert, 2009). Accordingly, self-compassion has been linked with enhanced distress-tolerance, clinically significant reductions in psychopathology, reflective and flexible perspective-taking, prosocial behaviour directed towards the self and others, and better adjustment to significant life stressors (e.g., infertility, cancer) (Mackintosh, Power, Schwannauer, & Chan, 2018; Macbeth & Gumley, 2012).

Compassion focused parenting can be understood in terms of how parents increase conditions for the maturation of these three types of affective functioning, and how they can blend together and support each other.

Currently this model of emotion regulation has not been applied to the field of parenting (Kirby, 2016), despite the benefits that can be gained from understanding their functions. For example, children receive report cards from school indicating their level of performance compared to other children (activates a competitive motive). If the child has performed 'average' or 'slightly below average' the child can feel 'anxious' about showing these results to their parents. If the parent was oriented towards a threat-based approach, the parent would then respond with frustration, and perhaps anger, in the hope that this will propel the child to study harder. This can indeed have the desired result, with the child foregoing other activities, studying harder, and achieving better grades the following semester. This can result in a short-term feeling of excitement and achievement for the child, which is then reinforced by the parent. However, taking a long-term view, the child then realizes in order to continue to receive this type of reinforcement he/she needs to continue to study hard otherwise their parent will be upset with them again (anxiety or threat-based). So we can see an interpersonal interaction between the parent and child of threat-drive-threat, a cycle, which is internalized by the child. Consequently, the child is learning to regulate their emotions through these two systems, which is then continued into adulthood, and can lead to a drive of perfectionism as the child strives for success. This is concerning, as when we are trapped between the threat and reward systems (competitive motives) this can often lead to a sense of failure and high levels of self-criticism, with an inability to self-soothe or be one's own secure base/safe haven (Gilbert, 2014).

If we consider children raised in family homes where they are the recipients of high levels of punitive parenting practices, like smacking, or at its worst, child maltreatment, that child would be operating from their threat-based/self-protect system, as they would be scared and fearful of their parents. These situations can lead to high levels of motive conflict for the child, as the caregiver has been the activator of threat, as opposed to the activator of affiliative/soothing behaviour. This has led some to theorize that children who live in family environments where they receive high levels of punitive parenting and child maltreatment, develop a self-identity where they are the 'cause' of the problem, and thus self-blame, as they believe that their care-giver would not engage in threat-based punitive practices unless they truly deserved them (Gilbert, 2014). Coupled with this is the key question, "Who do children turn to for affiliative connection and soothing when they are hit by their parents?" Perhaps, if the child is lucky, another family member, say a sibling or grandparent. Unfortunately, though, the child will often be left to themselves, alone, which can reinforce a core belief of rejection, unworthiness, and being unlovable. Moreover, threat can be activated from beyond the family home, with research by Horowitz, McKay, and Marshall (2005) finding that 50% of children from inner cities in the USA show high rates of posttraumatic stress disorder symptoms, due to their exposure to community-level stressors such as violence involving crime and weapons use. So it is critical to determine the environments in which children are being raised, as this is going to have life-long impacts on their ability to regulate their affect and form attachments with others (Mikulincer & Shaver, 2016; Pepping & MacDonald, this volume).

## Underpinning research: emerging evidence supporting compassion focused approach to parenting

Importantly there is emerging evidence in the field of parenting research supporting a compassion focused approach, indicating it is one which can be helpful not just for the parents, but also for the children. This research includes both cross-sectional survey design studies, along with experimental lab studies, as well as intervention evaluation of compassion-based approaches to help support parents.

To begin, Miller, Kahle, Lopez, and Hastings (2015) explored the relationship between compassion, autonomic nervous system activity, and parenting behaviours among 83 mothers during challenging interactions with their child. Mothers and their 3.5-year-old children were provided with two tasks. During the difficult puzzle task, mothers could give as much assistance to the child as required. During an origami task, mothers were instructed to provide verbal instruction only. Miller et al. (2015) found that greater self-reported compassion for one's child was associated with greater observed warmth, reduced observed negativity, and reduced harsh parenting.

Miller et al. (2015) utilized observational and physiological measures, supporting the conclusion that a compassion orientation protected against adverse parenting practices, even among those who experienced strong physiological stress. However, there has been little research exploring compassionate and self-image goals in relation to controlling and facilitative parenting. Our contention is that examining these links could provide insights into how motives influence parenting style, and thus offer a modifiable target (e.g., parent motivation) in parenting programs to help improve parent-child relating and positive childhood social, emotional, and behaviour development.

Based on this premise our team conducted research to examine whether goal orientation predicted parenting style (Kirby, Grzazek, & Gilbert, 2019). In this study, two goal orientations were examined, self-image goals (i.e., concerns with doing things wrong and being rejected) and compassionate goals (i.e., desires to be helpful), and whether they predicted psychological controlling parenting (i.e., controlling child's thoughts and self-expression) or facilitative parenting (i.e., warm and responsive). The study included 151 mothers, and the results found that goal orientation explained between 26% and 40% of the variance in parenting style, over and above child behaviour problems, parental mental health, and parental confidence. This finding is extremely important, as most parenting research indicates that it is the level of child behaviour which is most predictive of parenting style (Sanders & Mazzuchelli, 2019), whereas this research, the first to our knowledge, indicates that shifting motivational or goal orientation is a key pathway to parenting style.

Extending on these findings, Kirby, Sampson, Day, Hayes, and Gilbert (2019) examined the role that shame and compassion may play in texturing parenting style. The authors predicted that those parents who had high levels of shame (rank and self-image focused) and fears of compassion would engage in parenting styles that were both psychological controlling and dysfunctional. They conducted an online survey recruiting 333 parents of children aged between 3 and 9 years of age. Results from hierarchical and standard linear regressions found support for their hypotheses that shame and fears of compassion explain significant variances in parenting style, with models predicting 24% and 46% of the variance, respectively. These findings support past research indicating those who experience shame also find it difficult to experience compassion (Gilbert & Procter, 2006; Kirby & Gilbert, 2017).

Following on from this, Kirby, Grzazek et al. (2019) completed an experimental study where 198 mothers were randomly assigned to a compassion condition, a self-image condition, or a control condition (Kirby, Sampson et al., 2019). Mothers would then be presented with stressful child scenarios, for example a temper tantrum at the shops, and told to relate to the themselves with either self-image instructions (i.e., *we try to get our children to do things our way because we know what is best for them*) or compassionate instructions (i.e., *we all face challenges and setbacks and disappointments. Try not to be too hard on yourself*). The authors predicted the prompting compassionate goals would lead to reduced negative emotional reactions compared to the self-image condition, however there were no differences between the conditions. The authors concluded that brief instructions are not sufficient at shifting parental reactions to difficult child behaviour scenarios. Indeed, a greater level of intervention support is needed for parents.

In another study led by Kirby and Baldwin (2018), they examined the impact of a 15-minute Loving-Kindness Meditation as way to help improve parental reactions to difficult child behaviour. In this brief intervention study, Kirby and Baldwin (2018) examined the impact of Loving-Kindness Meditation (LKM) for parents of children 2–12 years of age (Kirby & Baldwin, 2018). LKM involves the repetition of short phrases (e.g., "*May you be safe, may you be peaceful*") towards oneself and others. A meta-analysis has found that LKM has significant moderate effects on compassion, self-compassion, as well as decreasing depression (J. Galante, I. Galante, Bekkers, & Gallacher, 2014; Hoffmann, Grossman, & Hinton, 2011). The Kirby and Baldwin (2016) study included 61 parents who were randomly assigned to receive LKM (15-minute guided audio) or a Focused Imagery (FI) exercise. The authors found that this brief intervention was sufficient in leading to emotional reactions that were different across the conditions, whereby in the LKM condition parents felt more calm and sympathetic towards the children, and less frustrated and angry. Moreover, LKM also improved the parent's level of self-compassion motivations compared to the FI condition. This study provides initial evidence for the use of LKM in a parenting context.

In an intervention design, we examined the feasibility and acceptability of a brief self-compassion intervention for mothers of infants (Mitchell, Whittingham, Steindl, & Kirby, 2018). The transition to motherhood can be challenging for many, especially when the mothering experience does not go as expected, which can lead mothers to feel guilty, ashamed, and distressed. For example, mothers can experience difficult and traumatic child birth (Soet, Brack, & DiIorio, 2003) and can have difficulty with breastfeeding attachment (Hall, McLelland, Gilmour, & Cant, 2014). The aim of this study was to support mothers experiencing this transition to motherhood. We developed brief online resources, which were informed by CFT, and included two videos on self-compassion meditation, as well as a tip-sheet. Overall, 262 mothers were recruited for the intervention, and results were examined pre-post, as there was no control comparison, which is a limitation of the study. However, the intervention found that it was able to significantly improve self-compassion, decrease posttraumatic symptoms, improve subjective breastfeeding experience, and improve satisfaction with infant feeding. However, the intervention was unable to change the level of shame experienced. Indeed, shame is an embedded and multifaceted experience, and a longer intervention would likely be needed in order to help mothers with the shame experience.

Finally, we recently embedded a compassion focused therapy module into the existing evidence-based parenting program (EBPP), Triple-P, in order to help Vietnamese parents who co-parent with their grandparents (Hoang, Haslam, Sanders, & Kirby, 2020). Past randomised controlled trial (RCT) research examining Triple P with parents and grandparents have found mixed findings, with positive outcomes for children, but never any improvements in the relationship between parent and grandparent (Kirby & Sanders, 2014; Leung, Sanders, Fung, & Kirby, 2014). Given these mixed findings, our research team decided to take a different approach and embed a compassion focused module to parenting to improve the parent-grandparent relationship, as past cognitive-behaviour communication strategies were not helping. Thus, we modified the existing Group Triple-P program, which includes eight sessions, each two hours, with the first four focused on 1) why children behave the way they do, 2) positive parenting strategies, 3) strategies to manage difficult behaviour, and 4) developing planned activities routines. The next four sessions are 20–30-minute phone calls with the parents to assist with the implementation of the new parenting routines. We then included an additional two sessions focused on building 1) compassion for oneself, 2) compassion for others when experiencing conflict, and 3) compassionate communication. These three modules included key CFT techniques, such as psychoeducation of the three-affect regulation model, soothing rhythm breathing, compassionate letter writing, and developing the compassionate-self meditation. One hundred parents were randomized in the intervention and compared to the control group, and for the first time, we found significant improvements in the parent-grandparent relationship, with reductions in conflict. Moreover, and possibly most importantly, we also demonstrated significant improvements in pro-social behaviour in children. Typically, EBPPs measure success through reductions of problematic behaviour, not increases in prosocial behaviour. Thus, this finding is particularly important.

### *Parenting increasing child's level of compassion*

An important rationale for the inclusion of the compassion focused approach in EBPPs is the aim of raising more compassionate children. Research has documented that children with empathic parents show more empathy themselves (Eisenberg, Fabes, Schaller, Carlo, & Miller, 1991). In contrast, the Making Caring Common Project at Harvard University surveyed 10,000 adolescents across the United States and found that 80% said that "achievement or happiness" is their top priority compared to 20% saying that their top priority is "caring for others" (Making Caring Common, Harvard, 2014). Moreover, the study found that youths were three times more likely to agree than disagree with the statement: "My parents are prouder if I get good grades than if I'm a caring community member." As a result, there is an important role for parenting interventions to help encourage compassion and caring behaviour in children and adolescents, as well as for school-based educational programs, which need to be developed, applied, and evaluated. Our initial research is suggesting that if you embed a compassionate module within existing EBPPs there is the possibility of significantly improving prosocial behaviour (Hoang et al., 2020), but more work is needed to replicate these findings.

## The transition from pure research to application

A key first step to help transition compassion focused parenting principles from pure research conditions in the lab, is to implement these approaches within existing evidence-based parenting programs. There are a range of parenting programs shown to be effective at reducing coercive parenting practices and reducing child problem behaviour (Sanders & Kirby, 2014). For example, the Triple P-Positive Parenting Program (Sanders et al., 2014) and the Incredible Years Program (Webster-Stratton, 1998) are two examples of programs that have had a significant impact on parenting practices and reductions in child behaviour. Both of these programs have been referred to as EBPPs (Sanders & Kirby, 2014), as there is a significant number of randomized controlled trials supporting their efficacy. According to a meta-analysis by Kaminski and colleagues (2008) the major components of EBPPs tend to be: 1) providing knowledge around positive parenting practices, 2) teaching parenting skills on how to relate positively to children, 3) teaching parents how to be consistent with discipline, and

4) providing opportunities for in vivo practice of these new parenting skills with the child. These components are informed predominantly from operant conditioning and a social learning theory model, and indeed, these EBPPs emerged in an era where social learning theory was the prominent approach to understanding child development (1970s–1990s). Therefore, EBPPs originated to target the treatment of childhood conduct problems, where compliance and reduction of externalizing problem behaviours were the goals of these intervention models (Kirby, 2016).

The previously described EBPPs (e.g., Incredible Years, Triple P) emerged during this period and are still the prevailing parenting interventions used and endorsed by organizations such as WHO and by evidence-based parenting lists (e.g., Blueprints for Healthy Development, www.colorado.edu/cspv/blueprints/). What has been remarkable is due to the evidence supporting these EBPPs, governments are starting to provide free access to these programs to all parents in a public health approach to supporting parents and family environments (Sanders & Kirby, 2014). However, although EBPPs reduce externalizing behaviour problems, their potential at improving positive childhood social, emotional, and behavioural interactions (e.g., considerate behaviour, turn-taking, gratitude, empathy, showing kindness) and improving childhood physiology (e.g., heart rate variability) remain largely unknown. This is where new insights from evolutionary psychology can be helpful.

## *Embedding a compassion focused parenting approach in EBPPs*

The impact and effectiveness of EBPPs could be improved through the adoption of a compassion focused parenting approach. The overall aim of compassion focused parenting is to create an internal secure-base/safe-haven in the parent or a 'Compassionate Mind' so that they can respond to parenting challenges as they arise at their compassionate best, as opposed to from a threat or defensive orientation. Our prediction is that this orientation in parents will help improve childhood social, emotional, and behavioural development. However, randomized controlled trials are necessary to empirically test this proposition. There are many potential ways to embed a compassion focused parenting approach in EBPPs, and we will outline a few possible pathways.

Although parenting can be extremely rewarding, parents can also struggle with finding emotional balance, and often parents indicate difficulties with failure, criticism, shame, and guilt concerning perceived parenting mistakes (Haslam, Patrick, & Kirby, 2015). This is where a compassion focused approach can be helpful, as CFT was developed to directly target high levels of self-criticism and shame (Gilbert, 2014), and there is evidence supporting the effectiveness of CFT (Kirby, 2017; Kirby, Tellegen, & Steindl, 2017).

One potential pathway in applying a compassion focused parenting approach to EBPPs is helping parents understand physiology and to try and facilitate affiliative emotional relating between parent and child. Thus the inclusion of the three circle model of emotion regulation in EBPPs will enable parents to understand the function of evolved emotion systems, so that they can gain insight into 'what sits behind' the interactions with their children and parenting partners (e.g., spouse, grandparent). The benefit of including the three circle model is that it will also enable a de-shaming and de-blaming process to occur for parents, as they begin to understand how they did not design the brain and body to function in that way (Kirby, 2016). In so doing, this process can start to facilitate a greater motivation for parents to take responsibility for how their affect regulation systems function in order to help their children's social-emotional development.

To provide a practical example on some possible differences between compassion focused parenting and typical evidence-based parenting programs, take the example of going shopping with a 4-year-old child. Going shopping with children aged 3–9 is often regarded as a stressful parenting activity. In most EBPPs the key would be to prepare in advance and engage in a technique approach where you might 1) have activities prepared for your child as you engage in the shop (e.g., child has their own shopping list), 2) go at an appropriate time of day rather than when you are in rush, 3) discuss ground rules with the child before going shopping (e.g., stay close to mom/dad), 4) ensure you praise good behaviour whilst shopping, and 5) let the child know what consequences there might be if he/she does not follow your instructions (e.g., quiet time). A compassion focused parenting approach would also engage in the same techniques; however, it would also focus on grounding behaviours for the parent. For example, before going shopping the parent might engage in soothing rhythm breathing – a technique which increases heart rate variability, so that the parent's vagal tone is strengthened before going into the threatening context (e.g., the shops). With the increase in vagal tone, parent emotional reactions to challenging child behaviour would be minimized, and parents can respond in more helpful ways, like remembering the planned routines as opposed to yelling or shouting at the child. The parent might focus on what 'green circle' strategies they might be able to do when stressed; for example, focus on body posture or tone of voice. Given the context of shopping is stressful, a compassion focused parenting approach would also aim to normalize this, and recognize that it is not the fault of the parent that it is stressful; indeed shops have many design features that aim to take advantage of children asking for chocolate or toys. A final aspect of a compassion focused parenting approach would be to consider how the parent is self-monitoring and judging themselves as they engage in this activity, paying particular attention to tone of inner voice. Indeed, activating a compassionate mind before going into the shops, one textured by the qualities of wisdom, strength, and commitment, would be key, and is the focus of compassionate mind training (Gilbert, 2009). These are just some small practical examples of what a compassion focused parenting approach would include.

Finally, a key theoretical component of EBPPs is to ensure the parent is taking care of themselves, as if the parent needs are not being met this impacts their ability to meet the needs of their children (Sanders & Kirby, 2014). A recent and significant finding in the parenting literature is that although children with empathic parents benefit significantly (i.e., experience less depression and less aggression) (Chase-Lansdale, Wakschlag, & Brooks-Gunn, 1995), this comes at a great cost for the parents. In two studies, researchers found that the higher the reported empathy of parents towards children (Manczak, DeLongis, & Chen, 2016) and adolescents (Manczak, Basu, & Chen, 2015), the greater the negative impact on the parents, specifically on inflammatory markers. The authors concluded that when children suffer psychologically, empathic parents' immune systems suffer. Thus, although parental empathy is beneficial for children, parents must also take care of themselves. Therefore, a compassion focused approach could be an avenue that could facilitate parenting self-care so that parents can best take care of their own needs and those of their children.

## *Public health approach to parenting: wide-scale compassionate action*

EBPPs help promote nurturing family environments, which provide the conditions necessary for children to thrive, yet so few parents participate in EBPPs. A recent population survey of parents showed that 75% of parents who had a child with an emotional or behavioural problem had not participated in a parenting program (Sanders, Markie-Dadds, Rinaldis, Firman, & Baig, 2007). If greater proportions of parents engaged in EBPPs, this would not only benefit the immediate family, but would also have a ripple effect by creating more compassionate environments for us to live in, as it would be treating and preventing suffering on a large scale. This requires adopting a public health approach to parenting (Sanders & Kirby, 2014).

Public health approaches to issues such as car safety (e.g., adopting the use of seat belts in cars), smoking (e.g., restricting smoking indoors, increasing taxes), and mass shootings in Australia (e.g., gun buyback, restriction and permits on gun ownership) have been able to prevent suffering on a large scale by reducing incidence and prevalence rates for car injuries, rates of smoking, and the number of mass shootings in Australia (Chapman, Alpers, & Jones, 2016). Thus, public health approaches to issues that treat and prevent suffering can be considered synonymous to wide-scale compassionate action. A public health approach to parenting has the potential to reduce prevalence and incidence rates of child maltreatment, which would be a compassionate act (Sanders et al., 2014).

There is initial support for such an approach, with the Triple P-Positive Parenting Program (Prinz et al., 2009). In a place-based randomized design population trial that spanned over two and a half years, 18 counties in South Carolina were randomly assigned to either the Triple P condition or to a care-as-usual control group. Interventions consisted of a media and communication strategy, parenting seminars, parenting groups, and individually delivered programs. Any parent could participate in any of the programs they wished, depending on their need and interest. Following intervention, the Triple P counties observed significantly lower rates of founded cases of child maltreatment ($d$ = 1.09; 16% lower than comparison counties, slowing the growth of cases), hospitalizations and injuries due to maltreatment ($d$ = 1.14; 22% lower than comparison counties), and out-of-home placements due to maltreatment ($d$ = 1.22; 17% lower than comparison counties).

This was the first time a parenting intervention had shown positive population-level effects on child maltreatment in a place-based randomized design. Importantly, this study targeted all parents, not just those at risk. These results demonstrate that adopting a public health approach, and making EBPPs accessible to everyone, reduces levels of child maltreatment. Moreover, such an approach is cost-effective, as every dollar invested in the Triple P program yielded a $9 return in terms of reduced costs of children in the welfare system (Aos et al., 2014). In addition, a public health approach to parenting also has the capacity to de-stigmatize and normalize accessing parenting support. One of the most overwhelming barriers is the stigma associated with engaging in EBPPs (Prinz & Sanders, 2007). A real concern expressed by many parents is the shame they experience if they enrol in an EBPP, with a belief that other parents and people will think, "They must be bad parents if they are doing a parenting program." This narrative is a problem, and it only serves to increase the suffering the parents and children might be experiencing. This is where the public health approach to parenting, a compassionate normalizing approach, becomes very powerful. The value of a population approach is that it can benefit everyone, avoids stigmatizing anyone, and can also attract widespread citizen support (Moffitt et al., 2011). This approach is also supported from an evolutionary perspective (Ellis et al., 2012), where there is a growing consensus that interventions aimed at promoting more positive strategies have long-lasting effects, as long as such interventions do not pull out only high-risk individuals, which may inadvertently confer their status as being problematic (Ellis et al., 2012).

## The impact of the research

We know EBPPs are helpful in reducing coercive parenting practices and reducing problematic child behaviours. But we can do more than that. Currently, parenting interventions are 'technique' oriented, aimed at reducing problematic behaviour (Mingebach, Kamp-Becker, Christiansen, & Weber, 2018), and are not grounded in the understanding of physiology and emotional function from an evolutionary perspective (Kirby, 2016). Our premise is that many of the techniques in EBPPs will remain the same (e.g., attention, praise), but the model of *how* to facilitate positive parent-child relationships will shift to focus on evolved caring motivational systems and affiliative emotion processing, which requires an understanding of the evolved processes involved in parent-offspring caring and physiological regulating systems. This is important because children are born prepared to respond to certain kind of stimuli provided by the parent such as voice tone, facial expression, and physical touch (Dunbar, 2010; Mikulincer & Shaver, 2016). These processes are conveying important information about the safeness and parental investment available to the child, and set the physiological infrastructures for social-emotional development (Mikilincer & Shaver, 2016). As Bowlby (1969) pointed out, the provision of a secure base and safe haven offers an evolved context for child development. Compassion is important because it brings a range of recently evolved social intelligence competencies such as empathy, mentalization, and self-other differentiation (Gilbert, 2014) that enables sensitive and physiologically wise parenting. Compassion focused parenting not only is motivated towards reducing suffering and threats in the child's environment but also providing the opportunity for exploration and social, emotional, and behavioural growth. These are facilitated when parents themselves feel secure. When parents feel threatened and uncertain they are more likely to engage defensively, responding potentially impulsively.

Thus, the compassion focused parenting approach focuses on a range of social intelligence competencies, such as empathy, distress tolerance, and clarity of the intention in one's parenting style. Not many parents wake in the morning with the intention to yell at their children or smack them for misbehaviour. Yet, when parents are stressed and children misbehave these are very common techniques parents will utilize in the moment (Prinz et al., 2009). This is typically a result of how the brain has evolved, as our threat system is the most dominant processing system (Swain & Ho, 2017). Importantly, this is not the parents' fault, as parents did not choose to design their brain in this way, one focused on threat processing. Thus, compassion focused parenting requires parents to understand how their brain functions, and how that will impact the interactions, relationship, and the development of their child's social, emotional, and behavioural growth.

## Lessons learnt

There is great potential for compassion to play a central role in EBPPs, but much empirical research is required to determine its efficacy and impact on a range of important family outcomes. When we started exploring the impact of compassion in families, we found it surprisingly difficult. Many EBPPs are relatively 'fixed', as they have been disseminated and implemented as part of child and parent services. Change takes time. We have been working over the last five years to build empirical support to justify the inclusion of compassion to help parents and children. There is an important distinction between evidence of process and evidence of outcome. There is a large body of empirical evidence indicating how compassion and self-compassion mediates, moderates, and predicts successful parenting and child outcomes – evidence of physiological processes, self-report, as well as observational. However, outcome research focuses on evaluations of 'programs' using RCT designs, and here is the difficulty, as RCTs are often expensive. To date, we have only been able to trial one RCT with an EBPP that embedded a compassion module, yet taking this research work and translating to changes in program materials, which are then integrated into training programs and disseminated, takes a long time. Although we agree evidence of outcomes using RCT designs is important, it is becoming more difficult to obtain necessary grant funding to conduct such trials using active treatment groups, for example Group Triple P compared to Compassion Focused Group Triple P. We are unsure on how to resolve this dilemma.

### *Future research*

In terms of future research areas that we believe are crucial steps forward in this field, we need to ensure measuring compassion is included as an outcome in EBPP evaluations. For example, the measurement of heart rate variability (HRV) will become central, and correlating HRV to parenting style and child social, emotional, and behavioural outcomes will provide greater insights into mechanisms underpinning parent-child interactions. In addition, there are many parents who do not respond to EBPPs (Sanders & Kirby, 2015), so could it be that non-responders to EBPPs have high HRV, indicating reduced vagal tone flexibility, indicating a reduced capacity to take on new parenting styles? Thus, would an approach that aimed to increase HRV make it more likely for these parents to feel a greater sense of safeness to adopt new parenting approaches and have less fears, blocks, and resistances to positive parenting practices? These are important questions that remain unanswered, but could have significant implications for the future success of EBPPs.

Self-report measures already exist, such as the Fears of Compassion Scale (Gilbert et al., 2010), and including these measures can also assist in determining whether compassion acts as a significant moderator or mediator to EBPPs, as determined by shift in parenting style and child social, emotional, and behavioural outcomes. Moreover, there are some parents who are non-responders to EBPPs (Maccoby & Martin, 1983), and a potential reason for this could be due to the parents own fears, blockers, and resistances (FBRs) to positive affiliative emotions and behaviours which they are confronted with when participating in EBPPs. Thus, an important area of research is to examine whether the inclusion of compassion helps address these FBRs (Kirby, Day, & Sagar, 2019) to help increase responsiveness and maintain parent participation in EBPPs. Compassion may also have differential impacts on certain parenting populations. For example, would compassion-based exercises in EBPPs have greater impact on parents of young children or teenagers? Or perhaps parents of children with long-standing difficulties, such as chronic health illnesses or clinical conditions such as autism or attention-deficit/hyperactivity disorder, may benefit most from compassion-based EBPPs. Or potentially it is parents with high levels of shame and self-criticism who stand to benefit the most from compassion based EBPPs.

A key future research question is to determine whether a compassion focused approach to parenting increases the efficacy of EBPPs when compared to existing interventions. In evaluations outcomes should not only be focused on short-term (e.g., pre-, post-, and six-month follow-up), but also longitudinal outcomes (5, 10, 30 years) to determine the impacts of compassion focused parenting. Multiple sources of assessment would be helpful to understand the impact of compassion focused parenting, so through observation of parent-child interactions, sibling-interactions, and physiological measurements (e.g., hear rate variability) of children and parents, as well as self-report scales.

## Concluding remarks

To conclude, with the advances in the understanding of how the brain functions and the importance of understanding evolved caring motivational systems and affiliative emotion processing, the next generation of EBPPs has an exciting future. Compassion focused parenting has the potential to help de-stigmatize and de-shame parenting experiences, helping parents with the rewarding and at times challenging experiences that occur when raising children. The further benefit of a compassion focused parenting approach is the hope that it will also raise compassionate children. In summarizing, Paul Gilbert (personal communication) provides a poignant insight into why this area of compassion focused parenting is so important:

> It is quite extraordinary that, given what we know about how early lives effect brain maturation and even genetic expression,

we have such limited resources dedicated to the desire for "every child to grow-up in a compassionate environment". This failure to grasp the size and nature of the problem, of "how children around the world are raised in appalling conditions", is probably humanity's greatest compassion failure!

## References

Aos, S., Lee, S., Drake, E., Pennuci, A., Klima, T., Miller, M., . . . Burley, M. (2014). Return on investment: Evidence-based options to improve statewide outcomes (Document No. 11–07–1201). Olympia, WA: Washington State Institute of Public Policy.

Biglan, A., Flay, B. R., Embry, D. D., & Sandler, I. N. (2012). The critical role of nurturing environments for promoting human well-being. *American Psychologist*, *67*, 257–271. doi:10.1037/a0026796

Bowlby, J. (1969). *Attachment and loss, Vol. 1: Attachment*. London: Hogarth Press.

Bugental, D. B., Martorell, G. A., & Barraza, V. (2003). The hormonal costs of subtle forms of infant maltreatment. *Hormones and Behavior*, *43*, 237–244. doi:10.1016/S0018-506X(02)00008-9

Carona, C., Rijo, D., Ssalvador, C., Castilho, P., & Gilbert, P. (2017). Compassion-focused therapy with children and adolescents. *British Journal of Psychiatry Advances*. doi:10.1192/apt.bp.115.015420

Chapman, S., Alpers, P., & Jones, M. (2016). Association between gun law reforms and intentional firearm deaths in Australia, 1970–2013. *Journal of the American Medical Association*, *316*, 291–299. doi:10.1001/jama.2016.8752

Chase-Lansdale, P. L., Wakschlag, L. S., & Brooks-Gunn, J. (1995). A psychological perspective on the development of caring in children and youth: The role of the family. *Journal of Adolescence*, *18*, 515–556.

D'Souza, A. J., Russell, M., Wood, B., Signal, L., & Elder, D. (2016). Attitudes to physical punishment of children are changing. *Archives of Disease in Childhood*, *101*, 690–693. doi:10.1136/archdischild-2015-310119

Dunbar, R. I. M. (2010). The social role of touch in humans and primates: Behavioural function and neurobiological mechanisms. *Neuroscience & Biobehavioral Reviews*, *34*, 260–268. doi:10.1016/j.neubiorev.2008.07.001

Eisenberg, N., Fabes, R. A., Schaller, M., Carlo, G., & Miller, P. A. (1991). The relations of parental characteristics and practices to children's vicarious emotional responding. *Child Development*, *62*, 1393–1408.

Ellis, B. J., Del Guidice, M., Dishion, T. J., Figueredo, A. J., Gray, P., Griskevicius, V., . . . Wilson, D. S. (2012). The evolutionary basis of risky adolescent behavior: Implications for science, policy, and practice. *Developmental Psychology*, *48*, 598–653. doi:10.1037/a0026220

Felitti, V. J., Anda, R. F., Nordenberg, D., Williamson, D. F., Spitz, A. M., Edwards, V., . . . Marks, J. S. (1998). Relationship of childhood abuse and household dysfunction to many of the leading causes of death in adults: The Adverse

Childhood Experiences (ACE) study. *American Journal of Preventive Medicine, 14*, 245–258.

Fogel, A., Melson, G. F., & Mistry, J. (1986). Conceptualising the determinants of nurturance: A reassessment of sex differences. In A. Fogel & G. F. Melson (Eds.), *Origins of nurturance: Developmental, biological and cultural perspectives on caregiving* (pp. 69–90). Hillsdale, NJ: Lawrence Erlbaum Associates.

Galante, J., Galante, I., Bekkers, M. J., & Gallacher, J. (2014). Effect of kindness-based meditation on health and well-being: A systematic review and meta-analysis. *Journal of Consulting and Clinical Psychology, 82*, 1101–1114. doi:10.1037/a0037249

Gilbert, P. (2009). *The compassionate mind*. London: Constable & Robinson Ltd.

Gilbert, P. (2014). The origins and nature of compassion focused therapy. *British Journal of Clinical Psychology, 53*, 6–41. doi:10.1111/bjc.12043

Gilbert, P., McEwan, K., Matos, M., & Rivis, A. (2010). Fears of compassion: Development of three self-report measures. *Psychology and Psychotherapy: Theory, Research and Practice, 84*, 239–255. doi:10.1348/147608310X526511

Gilbert, P., & Procter, S. (2006). Compassionate Mind Training for people with high shame and self-criticism: Overview and pilot study of a group therapy approach. *Clinical Psychology & Psychotherapy, 13*, 353–379.

Goetz, J. L., Keltner, D., & Simon-Thomas, E. (2010). Compassion: An evolutionary analysis and empirical review. *Psychological Bulletin, 136*, 351–374. doi:10.1037/a0018807

Hall, H., McLelland, G., Gilmour, C., & Cant, R. (2014). 'It's those first few weeks': Women's views about breastfeeding support in an Australian outer metropolitan region. *Women Birth, 27*, 259–265.

Haslam, D. M., Patrick, P., & Kirby, J. N. (2015). Giving voice to working mothers: A consumer informed study to program design for working mothers. *Journal of Child and Family Studies, 24*, 2463–2473. doi:10.1007/s10826-014-0049-7

Henri, J., Dionne, G., Viding, E., Vitaro, F., Brendgen, M., Tremblay, R. E., & Bolvin, M. (2018). Early warm-rewarding parenting moderates the genetic contributions to callous-unemotional traits in childhood. *Journal of Child Psychology & Psychiatry, 59*, 1282–1288. doi:10.1111/jcpp.12918

Hoang, A., Sanders, M. R., Haslam, D., & Kirby, J. N. (2020). The effectiveness of Group Triple P with a Compassionate Mind Training Module for Vietnamese parents and grandparents. Manuscript under review.

Hoffmann, S. G., Grossman, P., & Hinton, D. E. (2011). Loving-kindness and compassion meditation: Potential for psychological intervention. *Clinical Psychology Review, 13*, 1126–1132. doi:10.1016/j.cpr.2011.07.003

Horowitz, K., McKay, M., & Marshall, R. (2005). Community violence and urban families: Experiences, effects, and directions for intervention. *American Journal of Orthopsychiatry, 75*, 356–368. Retrieved from http://dx.doi.org/10.1037/0002-9432.75.3.356

Jackson, S., Thompson, R. A., Christiansen, E. H., Colman, R. A., Wyatt, J., Buckendahl, C. W., . . . Peterson, R. (1999). Predicting abuse-prone parental attitudes and discipline practices in a nationally representative sample. *Child Abuse & Neglect*, *23*, 15–29.

Kaminski, J. W., Valle, L. A., Filence, J. H., & Boyle, C. L. (2008). A meta-analytic review of components associated with parent training program effectiveness. *Journal of Abnormal Child Psychology*, *36*, 567–589. doi:10.1007/s10802-007-9201-9

Kirby, J. M., & Badlwin, S. (2018). A randomized micro-trial of a loving-kindness meditation to help parents respond to difficult child behavior vignettes. *Journal of Child and Family Studies*, *27*, 1614–1628.

Kirby, J. N. (2016). The role of mindfulness and compassion in enhancing nurturing family environments. *Clinical Psychology: Science & Practice*, *23*, 142–157. doi:10.1111/cpsp.12149

Kirby, J. N. (2017). Compassion interventions: The programs, the evidence, and implications for research and practice. *Psychology and Psychotherapy: Theory, Research and Practice*, *90*, 432–455. doi:10.1111/papt

Kirby, J. N., & Baldwin, S. (2018). A randomized micro-trial of a loving-kindness meditation to help parents respond to difficult child behaviour vignettes. *Journal of Child and Family Studies*, *27*, 1614–1628. doi:10.1007/s10826-017-0989-9

Kirby, J. N., Day, J., & Sagar, V. (2019). The 'flow' of compassion: A meta-analysis of the fears of compassion scales and psychological functioning. *Clinical Psychology Review*, *70*, 26–39. doi:10.1016/j.cpr.2019.03.001

Kirby, J. N., & Gilbert, P. (2017). The emergence of the compassion focused therapies. In P. Gilbert (Ed.), *Compassion: Concepts, research and applications* (pp. 258–285). Abingdon, Oxon: Routledge and Taylor & Francis.

Kirby, J. N., Grzazek, O., & Gilbert, P. (2019). The role of compassionate and self-image goals in predicting psychological controlling and facilitative parenting styles. *Frontiers in Psychology*, *10*, 1041. doi:10.3389/fpsyg.2019.01041

Kirby, J. N., Sampson, H., Day, J., Hayes, A., & Gilbert, P. (2019). Human evolution and culture in relationship to shame in the parenting role: Implications for psychology and psychotherapy. *Psychology and Psychotherapy: Theory, Research and Practice*, *92*, 238–260.

Kirby, J. N., & Sanders, M. R. (2014). A randomized controlled trial evaluating a parenting program designed specifically for grandparents. *Behaviour Research and Therapy*, *52*(1), 35–44. doi:10.1016/j.brat.2013.11.002

Kirby, J. N., Tellegen, C. L., & Steindl, S. R. (2017). A meta-analysis of compassion-based interventions: Current state of knowledge and future directions. *Behavior Therapy*, *48*, 778–792. doi:10.1016/j.beth.2017.06.003

Klevens, J., & Whitaker, D. J. (2007). Primary prevention of child physical abuse and neglect: Gaps and promising directions. *Child Maltreatment*, *12*, 364–377.

Leaviss, J., & Uttley, L. (2015). Psychotherapeutic benefits of compassion-focused therapy: An early systematic review. *Psychological Medicine*, *45*, 927–945. doi:10.1017/S0033291714002141

Leung, C., Sanders, M., Fung, B., & Kirby, J. (2014). The effectiveness of the Grandparent Triple P program with Chinese families: A randomized controlled trial. *Journal of Family Studies*, *20*, 104–117. doi:10.1080/13229400.2014.11082000

MacBeth, A., & Gumley, A. (2012). Exploring compassion: A meta-analysis of the association between self-compassion & psychopathology. *Clinical Psychology Review*, *32*, 545–552. doi:10.1016/j.cpr.2012.06.003

Maccoby, E. E., & Martin, J. A. (1983). Socialization in the context of the family: Parent-child interaction. In P. H. Mussen (Ed.), *Handbook of child psychology* (Vol. 4, pp. 1–101). New York, NY: John Wiley & Sons.

Mackintosh, K., Power, K., Schwannauer, M., & Chan, S. W. Y. (2018). The relationships between self-compassion, attachment and interpersonal problems in clinical patients with mixed anxiety and depression and emotional distress. *Mindfulness*, *9*, 961–971.

Making Caring Common Project, Harvard University. (2014). The children we mean to raise. Retrieved from https://mcc.gse.harvard.edu/reports/children-mean-raise

Manczak, E. M., Basu, D., & Chen, E. (2015). The price of perspective taking: Child depressive symptoms interact with parental empathy to predict immune functioning in parents. *Clinical Psychological Science*, *4*, 485–492. Retrieved from https://doi.org/10.1177/2167702615595001

Manczak, E. M., DeLongis, A., & Chen, E. (2016). Does empathy have a cost? Diverging psychological and physiological effects within families. *Health Psychology*, *35*, 211–218. Retrieved from doi.org/10.1037/hea0000281

Mann, M. (1986). *The sources of social power*. New York, NY: Cambridge University Press. Retrieved from https://doi.org/10.1017/CBO9780511570896

Maternal and Child Nutrition Study Group. (2013). Maternal and child nutrition: Building momentum for impact. *The Lancet*, *382*, 372–375.

Matos, M., Duarte, J., & Pinto-Gouveia, J. (2017). The origins of fears of compassion: Shame and lack of safeness memories, fears of compassion and psychopathology. *The Journal of Psychology: Interdisciplinary and Applied*, *151*(8), 804–819. doi:10.1080/00223980.2017.1393380

Mikulincer, M., & Shaver, P. R. (2016). An attachment perspective on compassion and prosocial virtues. In P. Gilbert (Ed.), *Compassion: Concepts, research, and applications*. London: Routledge.

Miller, J. G., Kahle, S., Lopez, M., & Hastings, P. D. (2015). Compassionate love protects stress-reactive mothers from fight-or-flight parenting. *Developmental Psychology*, *51*, 36–43. Retrieved from https://doi.org/10.1037/a0038236

Mingebach, T., Kamp-Becker, I., Christiansen, H., & Weber, L. (2018). Meta-meta-analysis on the effectiveness of parent-based interventions for the treatment of child externalizing behavior problems. *PLoS One*, *13*, 1–21. doi:10.1371/journal.pone.0202855

Mitchell, A., Whittingham, K., Steindl, S., & Kirby, J. (2018). Feasibility and acceptability of a brief online self-compassion intervention for mothers of infants. *Archives of Women's Mental Health*, *21*(5), 553–561. Retrieved from https://doi.org/10.1007/s00737-018-0829-y

Moffitt, T. E., Arseneault, L., Belsky, D., Dickson, N., Hancox, R. J., Harrington, H., . . . Caspi, A. (2011). A gradient of childhood self-control predicts health, wealth, and public safety. *Proceedings of the National Academy of Sciences, 108,* 2693–2698. doi:10.1073/pnas.1010076108

Porges, S. W. (2007). The polyvagal perspective. *Biological Psychology, 74,* 116–143. doi:10.1016/j.biopsycho.2006.06.009

Prinz, R. J., & Sanders, M. R. (2007). Adopting a population-level approach to parenting and family support interventions. *Clinical Psychology Review, 27,* 739–749.

Prinz, R. J., Sanders, M. R., Shapiro, C. J., Whitaker, D. J., & Lutzker, J. R. (2009). Population-based prevention of child maltreatment: The U.S. Triple P system population trial. *Prevention Science, 10,* 1–12. doi:10.1007/s11121-009-0123-3

Regalado, M., Sareen, H., Inkelas, M., Wissow, L. S., & Halfon, N. (2004). Parents' discipline of young children: Results from the national survey of early childhood health. *Pediatrics, 113,* 1952–1958.

Sanders, M. R., & Kirby, J. N. (2014). Surviving or thriving: Quality assurance mechanisms to promote innovation in the development of evidence-based parenting interventions. *Prevention Science.* Advanced publication. doi:10.1007/s11121-014-0475-1

Sanders, M. R., & Kirby, J. N. (2015). Surviving or thriving: Quality assurance mechanisms to promote innovation in the development of evidence-based parenting interventions. *Prevention Science, 16,* 421–431. doi:10.1007/s11121-014-0475-1

Sanders, M. R., Kirby, J. N., Tellegen, C. L., & Day, J. J. (2014). The Triple P-Positive Parenting Program: A systematic review and meta-analysis. *Clinical Psychology Review, 34,* 337–357. doi:10.1016/j.cpr.2014.04.003

Sanders, M. R., Markie-Dadds, C., Rinaldis, M., Firman, D., & Baig, N. (2007). Using house-hold survey data to inform policy decisions regarding the delivery of evidenced-based parenting interventions. *Child: Care, Health and Development, 33,* 768–783.

Sanders, M. R., & Mazzuchelli, T. G. (2019). *The power of positive parenting: Transforming the lives of children, parents, and communities using the Triple P system.* New York, NY: Oxford University.

Schore, A. (1997). Early organization of the nonlinear right brain and development of a predisposition to psychiatric disorders. *Development and Psychopathology, 9,* 595–631.

Seigel, D., & Bryson, T. P. (2011). *The whole brain child.* New York, NY: Bantam Books.

Soet, J. E., Brack, G. A., & DiIorio, C. (2003). Prevalence and predictors of women's experience of psychological trauma during childbirth. *Birth, 30,* 36–46.

Swain, J. E., & Ho, S. S. (2016). Parental brain: The crucible of compassion. In J. Doty & E. Seppala (Eds.), *Oxford handbook on compassion science.* New York, NY: Oxford University Press.

Swain, J. E., & Ho, S. S. (2017). Neuroendocrine mechanisms for parental sensitivity: Overview, recent advances and future directions. *Current Opinion in Psychology, 15,* 105–110.

Webster- Stratton, C. (1998). Preventing conduct problems in head start children: Strengthening parenting competencies. *Journal of Consulting & Clinical Psychology*, *66*, 715–730. doi:10.1037/0022-006X.66.5.715

World Health Organization. (2014). *Child maltreatment (Fact Sheet No. 150)*. Geneva: WHO. Retrieved July 21st, 2016 from www.who.int/mediacentre/factsheets/fs150/en/

# 4

# SHAME MEMORIES THAT SHAPE WHO WE ARE

*Marcela Matos, Stan Steindl, Paul Gilbert and José Pinto-Gouveia*

## The context of the research

Shame is a critical, socially focused experience affecting a sense of self, vulnerability to mental health problems, and social and moral behaviour. Shame is one of the most powerful, painful and potentially destructive human experiences (Kaufman, 1989; Gilbert, 2007a; Nathanson, 1994; Tracy, Robins, & Tangney, 2007). According to several theorists (e.g., Fessler, 2007; Gilbert, 2007a, 2019; Tangney & Dearing, 2002), shame is linked to social threat with a variety of possible primary threat emotions including anger, anxiety and disgust, and often with a sense of defeat, loneliness and disconnectedness. It has been clearly distinguished from other similar processes such as embarrassment and humiliation (Gilbert, 1998, 2019).

The potential for shame seems universal, although it can vary in terms of triggers, intensity and chronicity. There are three forms of shame (Gilbert, 2003, 2007a):

1 *External shame* relates to the sense of threat from judging that one is looked down upon and shamed in the mind of others, as well as the related experience of social diminishment. The focus of attention is external to self and on 'self in the mind of the other'. Coping efforts can be to escape or try to repair one's reputation (Sznycer et al., 2016). In a major meta-analysis, Kim, Thibodeau and

Jorgensen (2011) found that external shame may more powerfully effect mental health than internal shame. External shame is also linked to stigma and stigma consciousness (Pinel, 1999).

2 *Internal shame* relates to one's own self-judgement. Attention is internally focused on qualities of self that one judges to be inadequate or undesirable. Unlike external shame, internal shame is driven by self-criticism and internal processes of social comparison. Internal shame should be distinguished from self-blame; for example people can feel ashamed of things they are not responsible for, such as disfigurements (Gilbert & Miles, 2002).

3 *Reflected shame* relates to shame we can bring to others by association, or others can bring to us (e.g., parents can feel shamed by the actions of their children).

## Shame from an evolutionary perspective

Shame is regarded as genetically prewired, an affective response to social threats, including actual or potential loss of social status, acceptance or esteem, and corresponds to evolved behavioural adaptations that assist humans to address these threats and successfully navigate their social environments, enhancing their chances of survival and reproduction (Darwin, 1872; Ekman, 1992; Gilbert, 2007a).

The origins of shame are to be found in the evolution of hierarchical living where subordinates need to be wary of threats from dominant members (Gilbert, 1992, 1998). When threatened, subordinates express specific defences to reduce the attack from the dominant. These include eye-gaze avoidance, making the body smaller and reduced outputs, all of which are characteristic of shame (Keltner & Harker, 1998). These same evolved defences can be primed when people feel inferior or socially threatened or rejected. Hence, in so far as shame is related to relational issues, it is then a defence to social threat.

Social bonds are vital to human well-being and survival, and social threats make one at risk of being excluded, rejected, scorned, ostracized or even persecuted by others in the group, seriously compromising one's access to vital biosocial resources (e.g., food, support, protection) necessary for survival. Shame entails evolved systems to monitor and respond to these threats to the social self (Gilbert, 1998, 2003).

Shame motivational states (e.g., to hide, escape, appease or efforts to repair), nonverbal displays (e.g., eyes averted, head bowed, body slumped) and behaviours (e.g., submission, withdrawal) may function as appeasement strategies to reduce social conflict and restore social relationships (Fessler, 2007; Gilbert, 2007a; Gruenewald, Dickerson, & Kemeny, 2007; Keltner & Harker, 1998). Shame has an undeniable adaptive value to human psychosocial functioning and development, despite profound liabilities to mental and physical well-being (Gilbert, 1998, 2007a).

## *Psychological impacts of shame*

As an aversive and stressful experience that indicates threat to social relationships, shame can change one's mental state and prompt coordinated threat-related neuronal and psychobiological responses, with enduring consequences to cognitive and emotional processing and behaviour, damaging mental and physical well-being (Dickerson, Gruenewald, & Kemeny, 2009; Eisenberger, Lieberman, & Williams, 2003). Moreover, shame can form a part of one's self-identity as flawed, unlovable, inferior and a failure (Gilbert, 2007a; Tangney, 2003).

External and internal shame are central to psychological disturbance (e.g., Gilbert & Andrews, 1998; Tangney & Dearing, 2002; Tracy et al., 2007) and recognized as pathogenic and transdiagnostic processes associated with a number of clinical problems, including:

- Depression (e.g., Kim et al., 2011 for a review);
- Anxiety (e.g., Fergus, Valentiner, McGrath, & Jencius, 2010; Irons & Gilbert, 2005);
- Social anxiety (e.g., Gilbert, 2000; Grabhorn, Stenner, Stangier, & Kaufhold, 2006);
- Posttraumatic stress disorder (e.g., López-Castro, Saraiya, Zumberg-Smith, & Dambreville, 2019 for a review);
- Eating disorders (e.g., Blythin et al., 2018; Steindl, Buchanan, Goss, & Allan, 2017 for a review);
- Personality disorders (e.g., Brown, Linehan, Comtois, Murray, & Chapman, 2009; Schoenleber & Berenbaum, 2010);
- Psychotic disorders (e.g., Birchwood, Meaden, Trower, & Gilbert, 2002; Miller & Mason, 2005); and
- Psychopathy (e.g., Morrison & Gilbert, 2001).

Much still needs to be understood about the phenomenology of shame, how shame experiences are structured as emotional memories and the implications of these memories on psychological functioning and distress. The program of research summarized in this chapter adopts an evolutionary psychology approach and explores the nature of shame experiences and memories, and their effects on human suffering.

## Underpinning research

The program of research described later followed a series of key research questions:

1. Can shame memories function as autobiographical and traumatic memories, central to self-identity, and impacting current shame and psychopathological indicators?
2. Is there any specificity in the way shame traumatic and central memories affect psychological difficulties beyond their negative emotional valence?
3. Is there a role of attachment and affiliation on the structure of shame memories and their effects on psychopathology?
4. Are positive affiliative memories and compassion capable of buffering the negative impact of shame and shame memories on psychological distress?
5. Are early affiliative experiences, either shame or safeness memories, related to the origins of fears of compassion?
6. What are the defining phenomenological features of shame experiences?

### *The traumatic qualities and centrality of shame memories and psychopathology*

The program of research began by investigating the traumatic qualities and centrality to identity of early shame memories, and how these aspects of shame memories relate to current psychopathology. Many, but by no means all, shame memories will involve memories of an interaction, thus carrying memories of both the shaming actions of the other and their impact on the self (Kaufman, 1989). Shame experiences recalled from childhood and adolescence were found to be encoded in autobiographical memory and have traumatic qualities, eliciting intrusions, hyperarousal and avoidance symptoms. These shame traumatic memories were related to heightened proneness to external and internal shame, and to increased symptoms of depression, anxiety and stress in adulthood (Matos & Pinto-Gouveia, 2010).

The traumatic qualities of shame memories may engender a sense of ongoing threat to one's psychological integrity, resulting in individuals with shame memories feeling and believing they are seen by others as unattractive, inferior, defective, unlovable or inadequate, and judging themselves in the same negative and devaluing way. They are also more prone to experience feelings of defeat and threat. Moreover, these traumatic qualities moderated the association between current shame and depressive symptoms, in that individuals with higher traumatic qualities of shame memories have greater impact of external and internal shame on depressive symptoms.

Early shame experiences were also found to anchor self-identity, function as turning points in one's life narrative and cognitive references for attributing meaning to other experiences, and organize other memories and generate future expectations (Pinto-Gouveia & Matos, 2011). The centrality of shame memories may shape negative perceptions of the way one exists in the mind of the others (external shame) and one's own judgements of one's character (internal shame). Shame memories that are regarded as central to self-identity were significantly linked to heightened depressive, anxiety and stress symptoms in adulthood, independent of current external and internal shame effects on these symptoms.

Furthermore, the centrality of shame memories is related to the traumatic qualities of such memories (Pinto-Gouveia & Matos, 2011). Shame memories tend to become well-integrated in one's cognitive networks and form highly available reference points for organizing autobiographical knowledge and perceptions of the self and the world. This may influence their structuring as traumatic memories, incorporating intrusions, hyperarousal and avoidance symptoms.

Matos and Pinto-Gouveia (2018a) established that shame memories show autobiographical memory properties: elevated strength of recollection, vividness of visual and auditory imagery, heightened reliving and similarity of emotions, high story coherence, greater importance to self and lower rehearsal. Moreover, these autobiographical memory properties are enhanced in shame memories that function as traumatic and central to identity, and are associated with increased external and internal shame, and elevated symptoms of depression, anxiety and stress. This study revealed an integrative mediational chain model in which reliving of emotions, importance to self and rehearsal properties of shame autobiographical memory indirectly related to increased external and internal shame, and elevated depressive, anxiety and stress symptoms, through heightened traumatic qualities and centrality of shame memories.

Thus, these autobiographical memory properties confer a flashback quality to shame memories, which operate as conditioned emotional memories. When a shame memory is triggered one can return to the original shame experience, reliving its visual, auditory, language, cognitive and emotional components. This may elevate the shame memory's traumatic and centrality to identity features. Traumatic and central shame memories may engender and reinforce a sense of current threat to social attractiveness and psychological integrity, and impact one's sense of self as it exists in the minds of the others and in one's self, resulting in higher risk to experience symptoms of depression, anxiety and stress. In turn, elevated proneness to external and internal shame further increases one's vulnerability to feel defeated and threatened.

Matos, Pinto-Gouveia and Gilbert (2013) also found that external shame is especially associated with paranoid ideation whereas internal shame is especially related to social anxiety symptoms. When current external and internal shame were considered simultaneously, the degree to which shame memories have traumatic qualities and centrality to self-identity seems to be associated with increased paranoid anxiety, but not social anxiety. These results suggest that different psychological processes underpin these two distinct forms of social wariness. Paranoid anxiety may focus more on the malevolence of others' intentions towards the self and on how one exists in the minds of others, and traumatic and central shame memories may sensitize individuals to be socially wary and more prone to paranoid ideation. In contrast, social anxiety may be linked to feelings and beliefs focused on one's personal flaws, inadequacies and shortcomings.

Taken together, these findings extend existing models of shame, in particular the evolutionary biopsychosocial approach (Gilbert, 2007a), and current conceptualizations of autobiographical and traumatic memory (e.g., Berntsen & Rubin, 2007; Ehlers & Clark, 2000; Rubin, 2005), shedding light on shame memories as autobiographical and traumatic that can shape how we see ourselves, how we believe others see us and how we perceive others, as well as profoundly effect psychological well-being.

## *The role of attachment in shame memories and relationship with psychological distress*

Expanding upon the preceding studies and previous literature exploring the role early affiliative relationships play on psychological well-being (e.g., Belsky & Pluess, 2009; Cozolino, 2006; Gerhardt, 2004; Taylor, 2010; Schore, 2001; Siegel, 2001), results from Matos and Pinto-Gouveia (2014) and Matos, Pinto-Gouveia and Costa (2013) revealed that shame memories may function and effect psychological adjustment differently depending on whether they involved an attachment figure or other social agents.

In particular, Matos and Pinto-Gouveia (2014) found that the traumatic qualities and centrality of shame memories involving others from the wider social domain were more robustly associated with external shame, whereas these features of shame memories involving attachment figures were more strongly linked to internal shame and depressive symptoms. Furthermore, although shame traumatic and central memories involving others have an independent effect upon depressive symptoms, only shame memories involving attachment figures moderated the impact of current external and internal shame on depressive symptoms. Shame memories involving primary caregivers may amplify the impact of current shame feelings on depressive symptoms.

Results from Matos, Pinto-Gouveia and Costa (2013) showed that while rumination, thought suppression and dissociation mediated the relationship between shame traumatic memories involving others and depression, no mediator effect of these emotion regulation processes was found for shame traumatic memories with attachment figures, which directly effect depressive symptoms.

These data indicate that the quality and type of attachment relationships determine how shame experiences come to be structured as traumatic and central memories, and their association to current shame, emotion regulation processes and psychopathology vulnerability.

## *Memories of safeness as a protective factor*

Noting previous findings that positive affiliative memories, feelings of social safeness and connectedness foster resilience against adverse life events (Atwool, 2006; Cacioppo, Berston, Sheridan, & McClintock, 2000), the subsequent studies investigated the buffering effects of affiliative memories against the damaging impact of shame and shame memories on psychopathology.

Matos, Pinto-Gouveia and Duarte (2013) found that the effects of traumatic qualities and centrality of shame memories, and early memories of warmth and safeness, upon depressive symptoms may be mediated by internal shame. The internalization of shame traumatic and central memories, and lack of safeness memories, into a sense of self as unattractive, undesirable and inferior may elevate one's vulnerability to experience depressive symptoms. Conversely, recalling safeness as a child may lessen internal shame, and buffer against depression vulnerability. External shame, though strongly linked to internal shame, did not mediate these associations.

Matos, Pinto-Gouveia and Duarte (2015) went on to find that early memories of warmth and safeness seem to moderate the relationship between centrality of shame memories and depressive symptoms by attenuating their impact. This suggests that having a shame memory central to self-identity in the context of an early positive affiliative environment may provide opportunities for re-connectedness with others and buffer the negative impact of that shame memory on depression vulnerability. In the absence of positive affiliative memories, one may feel unsafe, alone and disconnected, and more vulnerable to the negative impact of central shame memories.

However, when shame memories have traumatic qualities their impact on depressive symptoms seems to be direct and not moderated by early affiliative memories. This implies that when early shame experiences have traumatic qualities, they engender a sense of enduring threat to one's sense of self and social status, activating the threat-protection system, which is not buffered by positive affiliative memories.

This study also showed that the protective effect of early memories of warmth and safeness, and the detrimental effect of shame memories central to identity on depressive symptoms, seem to operate through their effect on current feelings of social safeness and ability to use social relationships to soothe oneself when facing distress.

## *Compassion as an antidote to shame memories*

Research has revealed a protective role of compassion and self-compassion against mental health difficulties (e.g., Goetz, Keltner, & Simon-Thomas, 2010; MacBeth & Gumley, 2012; Zessin, Dickhäuser, & Garbade, 2015), and increasing evidence supports the effectiveness of compassion-based interventions, such as Compassion Focused Therapy (CFT), in the treatment of psychological disorders (Kirby & Gilbert, 2017), especially where shame and self-criticism are prominent (Gilbert, 2014; Kirby, Tellegen, & Steindl, 2017; Sommers-Spijkerman, Trompetter, Schreurs, & Bohlmeijer, 2018). We investigated this effect of compassion on the relationship between shame memories and psychological adjustment.

In a recent study, Steindl, Matos and Creed (2018) found that self-compassion mediated the effect of the traumatic qualities of shame memories and early memories of warmth and safeness on both depressive symptoms and safe positive affect. In two other studies, self-compassion was found to moderate the association between the traumatic features of shame memories and their centrality to identity, and eating psychopathology severity in women (Ferreira, Matos, Pinto-Gouveia, & Duarte, 2014), and to mediate the association between shame and safeness memories and depressive symptoms and internal shame in gay men (Matos, Carvalho, Cunha, Galhardo, & Sepodes, 2017). These findings suggest that competencies of self-compassion may act as an antidote against the deleterious effects of shame memories and a lack of memories of warmth and safeness on a range of mental health difficulties, and promote feelings of safeness.

## *Shame and lack of safeness memories at the root of fears of compassion*

Despite the robust evidence that cultivating compassion has powerful effects on a range of mental and physical well-being indicators (e.g., Barnard & Curry, 2011; Pace et al., 2008), research has shown that some individuals can develop fears of compassion, finding directing compassion toward themselves and others, and receiving compassion from others, difficult, aversive or threatening (Gilbert, McEwan, Matos, & Rivis, 2011; Rockliff et al., 2011).

Matos, Pinto-Gouveia and Duarte (2017) explored how early interpersonal emotional experiences might contribute to the development of these fears of compassion, finding that shame memories' traumatic and centrality qualities are associated with fears of compassion for self, for others and from others, whereas early memories of warmth and safeness are negatively related to such fears. Furthermore, fears of compassion for self and of receiving compassion from others mediated the effects of traumatic and centrality features of shame memories, and of early memories of warmth and safeness, on depressive and anxiety symptoms, and paranoid ideation. Hence, early shame experiences encoded as traumatic memories and central to self-identity, along with lack of experiencing warmth and safeness as a child, may be at the root of the development of fears of compassion for the self, for others and of receiving compassion from others, which in turn increases vulnerability to the effects of such early experiences on several psychopathological symptoms.

## *Shame memories phenomenology*

Further findings (Matos & Pinto-Gouveia, 2018b, 2018c, 2018d) extend the aforementioned research and underline the rich complexity of early shame experiences phenomenology using the Shame Experiences Interview (see Matos & Pinto-Gouveia, 2018b for a description).

Results showed that early shame experiences may take place within the family or the wider social domain, and typically involve being criticized, put-down, rejected, physically or sexually abused, bullied, negatively compared to others, feeling exposed or feeling reflected shame from family status or behaviour. Shame experiences of individuals with current mental health disorders included feeling neglected, deprived of love, care and support, or emotionally abused by attachment figures. These experiences may constitute threats to one's sense of self, social rank and relational bonds, and engender shame.

Early shame experiences entail rich phenomenological features, supporting both previous speculations (Kaufman, 1989; Nathanson, 1994) and the evolutionary biopsychosocial model of shame (Gilbert, 2007a). These experiences seem to be multifaceted, involving external and internal cognitive dimensions, and specific threat-related emotional, physical and behavioural components. At the heart of external shame experiences is a sense of self as unattractive and undesirable, unable to generate positive affect in the minds of others, who may condemn, reject, disengage or harm the self. This experience of the self as it exists for others may be internalized into derogatory self-evaluations and feelings that influence the self-experience and self-to-self relationship.

Shame experiences and memories are textured by a blend of primary defensive emotions, such as anxiety, anger, disgust or sadness. Shame experiences seem to be associated with defensive responses (e.g., submission, flight, escape, hide or sometimes fight). Such shame coping strategies may also involve internalized or externalized blame. These coping mechanisms following a shame experience seem designed to limit social damage, restore one's social image/reputation, de-escalate social conflict and repair damage to social bonds (Gilbert, 2007a; Keltner & Harker, 1998).

Shame experiences are common, though more frequent during childhood and adolescence, with shame episodes involving others from wider social contexts more often than those involving caregivers. Nonetheless, for some people, their most significant and difficult shame experiences are too painful to disclose and therefore kept secret.

The traumatic qualities and centrality of shame memories seem to be associated with the intensity of these phenomenological properties of early shame events, and are generally stronger in shame memories involving caregivers compared to those involving others. Distinguishing shame memories with caregivers versus other social agents does not so much involve the 'quality' or 'type' of their phenomenological features, but the intensity of the relationship between such features and the traumatic qualities and centrality of the memories. Our findings indicated that having an early shame memory that operates as traumatic and central seems to be related to current elevated levels of external and internal shame, higher negative social comparisons and increased psychopathological indicators, namely depression, anxiety, stress and dissociative symptoms.

Individuals with mental health disorders tend to present significantly higher levels of cognitive, emotional, physical and behavioural phenomenology of early shame experiences, negative impact on one's life, and traumatic, central and autobiographical memory properties, in comparison to individuals from the general population. In patients, associations between the phenomenological characteristics of shame experiences and traumatic qualities and centrality of the memory were also stronger. These data support shame processes and shame memories as ubiquitous. For some individuals, they can become extremely powerful and pathogenic, key to self-identity and psychological well-being, and on a continuum from lower level shame experiences common in the general population, to more severe levels present in clinical populations.

Further, patients more readily accessed general negative emotional memories than positive ones, whereas individuals from the general population access positive emotional memories more readily than negative ones. In contrast, patients' positive affiliative memories with attachment figures were less accessible and central to identity than general population participants, whose positive affiliative memories were more central to identity than shame memories. Access to warm and supportive, in contrast to shaming, emotional memories of the self-in-relationship-to-others may influence individuals' emotional and social responses to negative life events and, ultimately, vulnerability to psychopathology. Having access to early positive affiliative memories that become central to personal identity might foster feelings of social safeness and connectedness that promote affect regulation, soothing threat-related distress, and thus protect individuals against the detrimental impact of shame-related experiences and memories.

As a whole, these findings add to existing theoretical conceptualizations of shame and shame memories, and are incorporated in the evolutionary biopsychosocial model of shame (Gilbert, 2007a), as well as in current traumatic and autobiographical memory theories (e.g., Berntsen & Rubin, 2007; Ehlers & Clark, 2000; Rubin, 2005).

## The transition from pure research to application

Our program of research has implications for clinical intervention and prevention. We propose pathways that might increase one's vulnerability to psychological distress, and possible protective factors that might reduce the damaging impact of shame and shame memories.

Table 4.1 outlines recommendations for shame and shame memories assessment and intervention in a clinical setting. Following that are recommendations for prevention.

In terms of preventive actions, results indicate the importance of assessing and working with shame experiences early (i.e., childhood or adolescence) to prevent them developing traumatic qualities and centrality to self-identity and effect future emotional distress (Cunha, Matos, Faria, & Zagalo, 2012).

Recently, a Compassionate Mind Training (CMT) intervention, 'The Compassionate Schools Program', derived from the evolutionary model developed within CFT (Gilbert, 2010), has been implemented in schools in the UK and Portugal with teachers, other school professionals, children and parents. This program was based upon research with community populations that showed significant beneficial effects on a range of psychological and physiological well-being indicators of just two weeks of practising CMT (Matos, Duarte, Duarte et al., 2017; Matos, Duarte, Duarte, Gilbert, & Pinto-Gouveia, 2018). The Compassionate Schools Program has first been directed at teachers and non-teacher staff, with following research phases focusing on the impact of the 'Pupils and Parents' version of the program with students, and how teachers can guide students in developing compassion.

Findings from two pilot studies of the Teachers' Compassionate Schools Program (Matos, Albuquerque, Palmeira et al., 2019; Maratos, Montague et al., 2019) and preliminary results from two randomized controlled trials within Portuguese and UK schools (Matos, Albuquerque, Cunha et al.,

**TABLE 4.1** Recommendations for shame and shame memories assessment and intervention

| *Recommendations* | *Further considerations* |
| --- | --- |
| (1) Assess shame memories phenomenology, traumatic and centrality qualities, and current impact on external/internal shame, physiology and psychological well-being. Also assess positive affiliative memories. | The adapted Impact of Events Scale – Revised (IES-R; Weiss & Marmar, 1997), Centrality of Events Scale (CES; Berntsen & Rubin, 2007) and Shame Experiences Interview (SEI; Matos & Pinto-Gouveia, 2018b) are useful psychometric questionnaires and semi-structured interview for assessing shame memories. Positive affiliative memories are assessed via the Early Memories of Warmth and Safeness Scale (EMWSS; Richter, Gilbert, & McEwan, 2010). |
| (2) Assess the coping strategies and emotion regulation strategies used during and after the shame experience. | Certain behavioural responses may become prominent safety strategies activated every time the memory is triggered, and may maintain or aggravate current external or internal shame and/or psychological distress. Assess the emotion regulation strategies used to cope with shame traumatic memories, specifically rumination, thought suppression and dissociation, as they may affect the association between shame memories and psychopathology. |
| (3) Assess the frequency, and triggering cues, of shame memory reactivation. | Consider how often the shame memory is re-activated, as well as the common triggers. Also, consider evaluating the vividness of the memory, intrusiveness and flashback qualities, and associated re-experiencing and hyperarousal symptoms. |
| (4) Interventions should incorporate shame memories and positive affiliative memories. | Integrate both shame memories and memories of warmth and safeness into clinical case formulations and derive specific interventions as a part of treatment plans targeting them. |

(*Continued*)

**TABLE 4.1** (Continued)

| *Recommendations* | *Further considerations* |
|---|---|
| (5) Interventions targeting shame memories should incorporate compassion cultivation and trauma reprocessing. CFT can work with shame and shame memories via development of the soothing system. | Work with shame memories that are traumatic and central to identity, and significantly impact psychological distress, to lessen their traumatic nature and reconstruct their autobiographical meaning. A proposed intervention protocol for shame memories derived from CFT (Gilbert, 2009, 2010), and therapeutic interventions in traumatic memory and imagery re-scripting (Brewin, 2006; Clark & Ehlers, 2004; Lee, 2005; Wheatley et al., 2007), is given in Matos (2012). |
| (6) Interventions require careful management of the therapeutic relationship. | Beware of possible reactivation of shame memories in the therapeutic session (e.g., when the therapist shows affiliative emotions and care towards the patient, the high shame individual who has had few, or no, positive affiliative memories might become threat-activated and experience feelings of fear, anger, grief or disconnection; Gilbert et al., 2011). Assess and target possible fears of compassion in patients with traumatic and central shame memories. |

2019; Maratos, Sheffield et al., 2019) are promising and support the feasibility and effectiveness of this intervention in promoting psychological (e.g., increases in compassion, adaptive emotion regulation and positive affect, and reductions in shame, self-criticism, burnout and psychopathological symptoms) and physiological (i.e., reductions in systolic and diastolic blood pressure, total peripheral resistance) well-being in educators.

## The impact and legacy of the research

### *A comprehensive model of shame and shame memory functioning*

Building on the evolutionary biopsychosocial approach (Gilbert, 2007a), we propose an integrative and inclusive model of shame and shame memory functioning that incorporates the results of the program of research described earlier (see Figure 4.1).

Human beings are a highly social species whose survival and reproduction depend on our relationships with others. Social relationships are powerful physiological and psychological regulators. The quality of care we receive from the day we are born significantly effects gene expression, brain maturation, autonomic, neuroendocrine and immune functions, and influences the development of affect regulation systems (e.g., Belsky & Pluess, 2009; Cozolino, 2006; Gerhardt, 2004; Panksepp, 2010). So important are affiliative relationships to human survival and prospering that various evolved social motives guide us to form certain social roles, give ourselves social value, and understand and think of oneself in relation to others.

Shame is rooted in the thwarting of basic needs for social relationships. As shown in the model, shame experiences may therefore occur early in interactions within the family environment with attachment figures or the wider social domain. Shaming interactions in the family and with others may involve a range of socially threatening experiences (see Figure 4.1 for details), resulting in feeling unattractive and undesirable in the eyes of others, unwanted in the eyes of the self, vulnerable to social harm, and at risk of being ignored, demeaned, rejected, excluded, persecuted or even attacked by others (Matos & Pinto-Gouveia, 2014, 2018c; Matos, Pinto-Gouveia, & Costa, 2013).

Negative experiences of the self in the mind of others represent a social threat and block one's positive affect systems. Shame experiences seem to stimulate the threat system, and produce major changes in

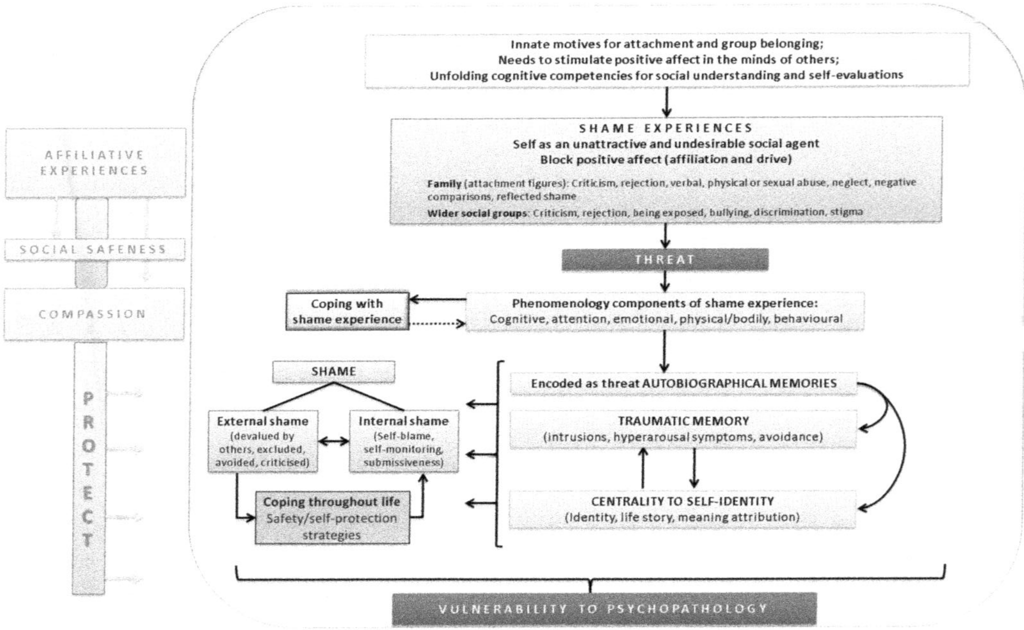


**FIGURE 4.1** An evolutionary and biopsychosocial model of shame and shame memory functioning

the drive and soothing systems. As social threats, shame experiences entail the separation and withdrawal from the 'shaming object', leading to the failure to attain biosocial motives and goals and access to resources. Setbacks related to social rank are likely to produce a loss of drive-based emotions. Simultaneously, shame experiences represent a block to the soothing system and potential 'soothing objects'. That is, shame-based threats are linked to inabilities to elicit acceptance and soothing from others, and undermine the development of feelings of safeness and connectedness, and self-soothing capacities. Therefore, shame experiences seem to engage all three affect regulation systems (Depue & Morrone-Strupinsky, 2005; Gilbert, 2010; LeDoux, 1998; Panksepp, 2010) and involve a triple problem: the social threat activating the threat system, the threat of separation and social setback linked to the drive system, and the threat of disconnection and lack of safeness linked to the soothing system, further triggering the threat system.

Thus, shame experiences constitute severe threats to one's social attractiveness, sense of self and social bonds, and seem to trigger specific patterns of threat-related psychobiological systems associated with amygdala sympathetic arousal. Once primed, the threat system directs attention, controls arousal and selects responses from a menu of evolved responses to threats, which might be experienced and expressed before conscious awareness (Gilbert, 2007b; LeDoux, 1998). So, shame experiences may operate through fast-track limbic-centred processes that automatically trigger a set of innate defensive responses (cognitions, attention, emotions, sensations, behaviours), which produce symptoms linked to the complex phenomenology of shame experiences. These seem to be richly multifaceted emotional experiences that comprise heightened defensive cognitive/attentional, emotional, physical/bodily and behavioural components (Matos & Pinto-Gouveia, 2018c).

In terms of cognitive and attentional focus, at the centre of any shame experience is a sense of external shame, usually accompanied by inwardly focused attention, thoughts and feelings around a sense of internal shame. Shame fuses with, and is textured by, a blend of primary defensive emotions (e.g., anxiety, anger, disgust, sadness), and a host of defensive physical and behavioural responses are triggered. These typically involve high levels of submissive and flight responses (e.g., averted eye gaze, head down, slumped posture, withdrawal, escape, inhibition), but also lower levels of fear bodily responses (e.g., body tension, heart racing) and defensive fight responses (e.g., externalizing anger, counter-attacking), as well as other specific action tendencies to hide, conceal, escape, submit or redo the situation (Matos & Pinto-Gouveia, 2018c). These physical and behavioural displays may be related to the rapid onset of basic submissive-flight defensive responses, akin to subordination displays in primates, and serving appeasement and social conflict de-escalation functions (Gilbert, 2007a; Gilbert & Andrews, 1998; Keltner & Harker, 1998).

Also in the model are defensive coping strategies usually triggered in the aftermath of a shame event to deal with the shame experience symptomatology, including those responses described earlier as well as the internalization or externalization of blame (Matos & Pinto-Gouveia, 2018d). These coping strategies may act to limit social damage, restore social image/reputation, de-escalate social conflict and mitigate damage to relational bonds (Gilbert, 2007a; Keltner & Harker, 1998). Although designed to deal with, and lessen, social threats, these defensive coping strategies may intensify shame phenomenological symptoms and aggravate the experience of threat.

Thus, intense and painful multifaceted shame experiences may lay down affect-based memories of the self-in-relationship-to-others, which are encoded autobiographically as emotional memories of threat. Such threat autobiographical memories tend to be associated with greater vividness of recollection and imagery, reliving and similarity of emotions, story coherence and importance to self, and lower rehearsal (Matos & Pinto-Gouveia, 2018a, 2018d).

Furthermore, these shame autobiographical memories have traumatic qualities, including intrusions, hyperarousal and avoidance (Matos & Pinto-Gouveia, 2010, 2018a, 2018d; Matos, Pinto-Gouveia, & Duarte, 2012, 2013), engendering current threat to one's sense of self and psychological integrity, rendering one to feel inferior, defective, powerless and socially unattractive. This ongoing threat to one's social self may contribute to threat-based attentional, emotional and cognitive processing (Ehlers & Clark, 2000; Harman & Lee, 2010).

These shame memories can become central to self-identity, viewed as turning points in one's life story, and forming highly available reference points to attribute meaning to past, current and future experiences (Pinto-Gouveia & Matos, 2011; Matos & Pinto-Gouveia, 2018d; Matos et al., 2012, 2013), becoming a central point around which the sense of self becomes organized. Shame memories construed as central and traumatic may operate as self-defining memories in the self-memory system (Berntsen & Rubin, 2007; Conway, 2005) and influence behaviour and personal goals (McAdams, Josselson, & Lieblich, 2006; Sutin & Robins, 2008).

The more traumatic the shame memory, the more central to identity it may become. The more central and well-integrated in one's cognitive networks the shame memory, the more it may be structured as traumatic (Pinto-Gouveia & Matos, 2011). The degree to which shame memories are traumatic and central to identity seems to be associated with the robustness of autobiographical memory properties (Matos & Pinto-Gouveia, 2018a), and the intensity of the threat-related phenomenological components of the shame experience itself (Matos & Pinto-Gouveia, 2018c, 2018d).

Therefore, shame memories seem to be embedded in the threat system and operate through specific traumatic memory systems and body-wide physiological systems (e.g., amygdala, subcortical brain areas) linked to conditioning and to the recreation of 'whole body effects' when primed (Brewin, 2006; Gilbert, 2007b; Rothschild, 2000). These heightened emotional memories of threat may work at implicit levels and influence psychobiological response patterns that guide emotional and cognitive processing, basic social engagement orientation and protection-safety strategies. Because these shame memories may operate as conditioned emotional memories of threat, every time they are triggered the original multi-textured emotional experience and psychobiological response patterns may be re-activated. So, the re-emergence of these emotional memories can change one's brain states (Brewin, 2006). In fact, these autobiographical memories may be strengthened by their persistent reactivation and by other shame experiences. They can become highly accessible, aversive emotional memories, easily triggered by events that threaten one's social attractiveness or social bonds (Matos & Pinto-Gouveia, 2018c, 2018d).

In addition, these shame memory scripts may shape the emotional foundations for negative internal working models of self and others, and integrate interpersonal schema (Baldwin, 2005; Gilbert, 2007b; Mikulincer & Shaver, 2004). As outlined in the model, shame memories influence how individuals perceive themselves as 'existing in the minds of the others' and how they see and judge themselves. Thus, shame memories seem to be associated with elevated proneness to external shame later in life and can become the basis for derogatory self-experience and self-evaluations, increasing proneness to internal shame (Matos & Pinto-Gouveia, 2010, 2014, 2018a, 2018d; Matos et al., 2012, 2013; Pinto-Gouveia & Matos, 2011).

Given shame memories and external shame activate defensive coping strategies to deal with social threat, one of these defensive manoeuvres may be to internalize shame into an enduring and global sense of self-condemnation. This involves high levels of self-monitoring, self-attribution and self-blame, and submissiveness aimed at appeasing and minimizing harm from others (Matos & Pinto-Gouveia, 2018d; Matos, Pinto-Gouveia, & Gilbert, 2013; Matos, Pinto-Gouveia, & Duarte, 2013). There are, however, other safety and self-protection strategies individuals may adopt during life to cope with shame, or to limit harmful shame/threat-based events (e.g., avoiding potential shame-eliciting situations, compensating and proving the self as worthy and competing to avoid inferiority, or externalizing shame as humiliation and defensive-fight responding; Matos & Pinto-Gouveia, 2018d).

As outlined at the bottom of the model, external and internal shame and shame memories are associated with increased vulnerability to psychopathology. In particular, shame traumatic and central memories have a unique effect in elevating vulnerability to psychological difficulties, such as depression, anxiety and stress, paranoid and social anxiety, and eating psychopathology (Cunha et al., 2012; Matos & Pinto-Gouveia, 2010, 2014, 2018a, 2018d; Matos et al., 2012, 2013; Matos, Pinto-Gouveia, & Costa, 2013; Matos, Pinto-Gouveia, & Duarte, 2013; Matos, Ferreira, Pinto-Gouveia, & Duarte, 2015; Pinto-Gouveia & Matos, 2011). Moreover, the traumatic, centrality to identity and autobiographical properties of shame memories tend to be elevated in people suffering from mental health disorders (e.g., depression, anxiety disorders, eating disorders, personality disorders; Matos & Pinto-Gouveia, 2018c, 2018d), and shame traumatic and central memories seem to intensify and strengthen the effect of external and internal shame on psychopathology vulnerability (Cunha et al., 2012; Matos & Pinto-Gouveia, 2010; Matos et al., 2012; Pinto-Gouveia & Matos, 2011).

Shame memories' effect on psychopathological symptoms seems to operate through their impact on elevating shame proneness, especially internal shame. Internalizing shame memories is critical in increasing vulnerability to enter defeat emotional states in face of adverse life events (Cunha et al., 2012; Matos & Pinto-Gouveia, 2018a; Matos, Pinto-Gouveia, & Duarte, 2013).

A key aspect to this model is the role of affiliative relationships and compassion in buffering and healing shame and shame memories. Affiliative relationships may lay down positive emotional memories of the self-in-relationship-to-others that provide a source of social safeness and connectedness and enable adaptive affect regulation through access to soothing objects. These offer opportunities to repair shame, self-soothe distress and regulate arousal caused by threat. So, they can protect against the effects of shame and shame memories at all levels of the model. Having positive affiliative memories that are accessible and central lessens the intensity of the symptoms of shame experiences, buffers the traumatic features and centrality to self-identity of shame memories and is related to fewer mental health difficulties (Matos & Pinto-Gouveia, 2018d; Matos, Ferreira et al., 2015).

In addition, compassion, particularly one's competencies for self-compassion in the face of life difficulties, may protect against the toxic effects of shame memories on psychological adjustment and promote positive affect (Matos, Carvalho et al., 2017; Steindl et al., 2018). Self-compassion may help down-regulate threat system activation in the face of shame memories by activating the soothing system. While competencies for self-compassion and receiving compassion from others may be inhibited by early experiences of shame and related threat system activation, they may be facilitated by early experiences of warmth and safeness and soothing system activation (Matos, Duarte, & Pinto-Gouveia, 2017; Steindl et al., 2018). One's capacity and openness to be the recipient of compassion from oneself or from others may emerge from early emotional experiences of being cared for and nurtured as a child, as these are thought to promote the development of one's soothing system and capacities for self-soothing (Gilbert, 2009; Matos, Duarte et al., 2017).

## Lessons learnt

The results of this program of research have been comprehensive and promising, and there has been a number of key lessons learnt along the way. One important difficulty encountered in the research is the predominance of cross-sectional design and the correlational nature of the data, which precludes drawing robust causal conclusions. Disentangling the circularity of the data can also pose difficulties, given that alternative conclusions might be derived from the same results (e.g., current emotional states might influence the degree to which shame memories are recollected as traumatic and central). Longitudinal and experimental designs will help to clarify the causal relations between the variables and the stability of the findings across time.

Research to date has been largely based on retrospective self-report, raising the issue of the accuracy and reliability of those recollections and social desirability. Retrospective recall data are considered generally stable, accurate and reliable (Brewin & Holmes, 2003), and a major strength of this research was the development and use of the SEI to assess shame memories phenomenology, which also corroborated the findings derived from self-report data adding further support to the validity of the findings.

Generally speaking, the research has used convenient samples, largely female, collected from general community, student and clinical populations. This lack of randomization may constrain the generalization of results to other populations. However, we have learnt that men and women may be equally affected by shame and no significant differences between these genders regarding shame and shame memories were found. It will be important to replicate these results using more equal samples. Ethnicity and age were not explored in regard to shame and shame memories and could be investigated in future studies. Also, studies have shown that the centrality of shame memories may change across the life span (Rubin & Berntsen, 2009).

One invaluable aspect of our program of research is the examination of clinical and non-clinical samples, with both similarities and differences across these samples being found. Further investigation in clinical populations is needed, such as investigating whether shame memories differ according to specific clinical groups; however it is important to note that shame and shame memories are present at clinical and non-clinical levels and are transdiagnostic processes (Matos & Pinto-Gouveia, 2018c, 2018d).

Recent social neuroscience research has shown that psychological sensitivity to stressful life events is influenced by gene-environment interactions and genetic variation (Belsky & Pluess, 2009; Caspi & Moffitt, 2006). Early stressful social environments can affect biological stress regulatory systems (Taylor, Lerner, Sage, Lehman, & Seeman, 2004) and influence mechanisms by which the brain manages stress (Taylor, Eisenberger, Saxbe, Lehman, & Lieberman, 2006), and affect the expression of genes and lead to epigenetic modifications, which negatively influence several mental and physical health outcomes (Kupfer, Frank, & Phillips, 2011; Taylor, 2010; Taylor et al., 2006; Tyrka, Price, Marsit, Walters, & Carpenter, 2012). We are currently investigating how shame experiences in early life influence epigenetic mechanisms, and how these processes influence vulnerability to psychopathology.

We are also interested to investigate how shame and shame memories are expressed and affect neurobiological stress systems. Studies could explore how shame memories trigger the threat system by examining specific neurophysiological correlates, such as cortisol, heart rate variability or fMRI brain activity, associated with the primed shame memories or with the activation of shame.

Importantly, our research has begun to explore the processes through which shame and shame memories can be healed, and whether compassion or self-compassion might protect against their pathogenic effects. We are carrying out experimental studies to test the effect of compassion focused (Gilbert, 2009, 2010) versus mindfulness-based (Kabat-Zinn, 1990; Segal, Teasdale, & Williams, 2004) interventions on mitigating the traumatic nature and centrality of shame memories and their impact on psychopathology. We are also investigating whether a compassion focused intervention developing the soothing system and cultivating of compassion competencies would be related to the activation of safeness-related physiological patterns and the decrease of threat-related biomarkers, influence epigenetic mechanisms related to stress and affiliation, and buffer the detrimental effects of shame memories, promoting mental and physical well-being.

## Summary

Shame can be an overwhelming emotional experience, embodying profound threats to the social self. From early in life, shame experiences can tear the fibres of one's being by damaging relational bonds in the social world. Shame experiences can leave deep scars in the self and be encoded in our autobiographical memory as powerful traumas, damaging one's most cherished and inner sense of identity, and influencing one's psychological well-being throughout life.

The results of this program of research shed light towards our further understanding of the rich complexity of shame and shame memories, and their potential pathogenic effects on mental well-being. We hope these findings will inspire future research to advance our knowledge of these processes and improve clinical interventions with individuals suffering from shame-related difficulties.

## References

Atwool, N. (2006). Attachment and resilience: Implications for children in care. *Child Care in Practice*, *12*, 315–330. doi:10.1080/13575270600863226

Baldwin, M. W. (Ed.). (2005). *Interpersonal cognition*. New York, NY: Guilford Press.

Barnard, L., & Curry, J. (2011). Self-compassion: Conceptualizations, correlates and interventions. *Review of General Psychology*, *15*(4), 289–303.

Belsky, J., & Pluess, M. (2009). Beyond diathesis stress: Differential susceptibility to environmental influences. *Psychological Bulletin*, *135*, 885–908. doi:10.1037/a0017376

Berntsen, D., & Rubin, D. C. (2007). When a trauma becomes a key to identity: Enhanced integration of trauma memories predicts posttraumatic stress disorder symptoms. *Applied Cognitive Psychology*, *21*, 417–431. doi:10.1002/acp.1290

Birchwood, M., Meaden, A., Trower, P., & Gilbert, P. (2002). Shame, humiliation and entrapment in psychosis: A social rank theory approach to cognitive intervention with voices and delusions. In A. P. Morrison (Ed.), *A casebook of cognitive therapy for psychosis* (pp. 108–131). London: Brunner-Routledge.

Blythin, S. P., Nicholson, H. L., Macintyre, V. G., Dickson, J. M., Fox, J. R., & Taylor, P. J. (2018). Experiences of shame and guilt in anorexia and bulimia nervosa: A systematic review. *Psychology and Psychotherapy: Theory, Research and Practice*. doi:10.1111/papt.12198

Brewin, C. (2006). Understanding cognitive behaviour therapy: A retrieval competition account. *Behaviour Research and Therapy*, *44*, 765–784.

Brewin, C. R., & Holmes, E. A. (2003). Psychological theories of posttraumatic stress disorder. *Clinical Psychology Review*, *23*, 339–376.

Brown, M. Z., Linehan, M. M., Comtois, K. A., Murray, A., & Chapman, A. L. (2009). Shame as a prospective predictor of self-inflicted injury in borderline personality disorder: A multi-modal analysis. *Behavior Research and Therapy*, *47*(10), 815–822.

Cacioppo, J. T., Berston, G. G., Sheridan, J. F., & McClintock, M. K. (2000). Multilevel integrative analysis of human behavior: Social neuroscience and the complementing nature of social and biological approaches. *Psychological Bulletin*, *126*, 829–843.

Caspi, A., & Moffitt, T. E. (2006). Gene-environment interactions in psychiatry: Joining forces with neuroscience. *Nature Reviews Neuroscience*, *7*, 583–593.

Clark, D. M., & Ehlers, A. (2004). Post-traumatic stress disorders from cognitive theory to therapy. In R. L. Leahy (Ed.), *Contemporary cognitive therapy: Theory, research, and practice* (pp. 141–160). New York, NY: Guilford Press.

Conway, M. A. (2005). Memory and the self. *Journal of Memory and Language*, *53*, 594–628.

Cozolino, L. (2006). *The neuroscience of human relationships: Attachment and the developing brain*. New York, NY: W.W. Norton & Company.

Cunha, M., Matos, M., Faria, D., & Zagalo, S. (2012). Shame memories and psychopathology in adolescence: The mediator effect of shame. *International Journal of Psychology and Psychological Therapy*, *12*(2), 203–218.

Darwin, C. (1872). *The expression of emotions in man and animals*. New York, NY: Philosophical Library.

Depue, R. A., & Morrone-Strupinsky, J. V. (2005). A neurobehavioral model of affiliative bonding: Implications for conceptualizing a human trait of affiliation. *Behavioral and Brain Sciences*, *28*, 313–395.

Dickerson, S. S., Gruenewald, T. L., & Kemeny, M. E. (2009). Psychobiological responses to social self threat: Functional or detrimental? *Self and Identity*, *8*, 270–285.

Ehlers, A., & Clark, D. (2000). A cognitive model of posttraumatic stress disorder. *Behaviour Research and Therapy*, *38*(4), 319–345. doi:10.1016/S0005-7967(99)00123-0

Eisenberger, N. I., Lieberman, M. D., & Williams, K. D. (2003). Does rejection hurt? An fMRI study of social exclusion. *Science*, *302*, 290–292.

Ekman, P. (1992). An argument for basic emotions. *Cognition and Emotion*, *6*, 169–200.

Fergus, T. A., Valentiner, D. P., McGrath, P. B., & Jencius, S. (2010). Shame- and guilt-proneness: Relationships with anxiety disorder symptoms in a clinical sample. *Journal of Anxiety Disorders*, *24*, 811–815.

Ferreira, C., Matos, M., Pinto-Gouveia, J., & Duarte, C. (2014). Shame memories and eating psychopathology: The buffering effect of self-compassion. *European Eating Disorders Review*, *22*(6), 487–494. doi:10.1002/erv.2322

Fessler, D. M. T. (2007). From appeasement to conformity: Evolutionary and cultural perspectives on shame, competition, and cooperation. In J. Tracy, R. Robins, & J. Tangney (Eds.), *Self-conscious emotions: Theory and research* (2nd ed., pp. 174–193). New York, NY: Guilford Press.

Gerhardt, S. (2004). *Why love matters: How affection shapes a baby's brain*. London: Brunner-Routledge.

Gilbert, P. (1992). *Depression: The evolution of powerlessness*. Hove: Lawrence Erlbaum Associates.

Gilbert, P. (1998). What is shame? Some core issues and controversies. In P. Gilbert & B. Andrews (Eds.), *Shame: Interpersonal behaviour, psychopathology and culture* (pp. 3–36). New York, NY: Oxford University Press.

Gilbert, P. (2000). The relationship of shame, social anxiety and depression: The role of the evaluation of social rank. *Clinical Psychology and Psychotherapy*, *7*, 174–189.

Gilbert, P. (2003). Evolution, social roles and the differences in shame and guilt. *Social Research*, *70*, 1205–1230.

Gilbert, P. (2007a). The evolution of shame as a marker for relationship security. In J. L. Tracy, R. W. Robins, & J. P. Tangney (Eds.), *The self-conscious emotions: Theory and research* (pp. 283–309). New York, NY: Guilford Press.

Gilbert, P. (2007b). *Psychotherapy and counselling for depression* (3rd ed.). London: Sage.

Gilbert, P. (2009). *The compassionate mind: A new approach to life's challenges*. London: Constable & Robinson Ltd.

Gilbert, P. (2010). *Compassion focused therapy: Distinctive features*. London: Routledge.

Gilbert, P. (2014). The origins and nature of compassion focused therapy. *British Journal of Clinical Psychology*, *53*(1), 6–41.

Gilbert, P. (2019). Distinguishing shame, humiliation and guilt: An evolutionary functional analysis and compassion focused interventions. In C.-H. Mayer & E. Vanderheiden (Eds.), *The bright side of shame* (pp. 413–432). New York, NY: Springer.

Gilbert, P., & Andrews, B. (Eds.). (1998). *Shame: Interpersonal behavior, psychopathology and culture*. New York, NY: Oxford University Press.

Gilbert, P., McEwan, K., Matos, M., & Rivis, A. (2011). Fear of compassion: A study of psychological processes that block compassion. *Psychology and Psychotherapy: Theory, Research and Practice*, *84*, 239–255. doi:10.1348/147608310X526511

Gilbert, P., & Miles, J. (2002). *Body shame: Conceptualizations, research & treatment*. London: Brunner-Routledge.

Goetz, J., Keltner, D., & Simon-Thomas, E. (2010). Compassion: An evolutionary analysis and empirical review. *Psychological Bulletin*, *136*(3), 351–374.

Grabhorn, R., Stenner, H., Stangier, U., & Kaufhold, J. (2006). Social anxiety in anorexia and bulimia nervosa: The mediating role of shame. *Clinical Psychology and Psychotherapy*, *13*, 12–19.

Gruenewald, T. L., Dickerson, S. S., & Kemeny, M. E. (2007). A social function for the self-conscious emotions: Social-self preservation theory. In J. Tracy, R. Robins, & J. Tangney (Eds.), *Self-conscious emotions: Theory and research* (2nd ed., pp. 68–87). New York, NY: Guilford Press.

Harman, R., & Lee, D. (2010). The role of shame and self-critical thinking in the development and maintenance of current threat in post-traumatic stress disorder. *Clinical Psychology & Psychotherapy*, *17*, 13–24. doi:10.1002/cpp.636

Irons, C., & Gilbert, P. (2005). Evolved mechanisms in adolescent anxiety and depression symptoms: The role of attachment and social rank systems. *Journal of Adolescence*, *28*, 325–341.

Kabat-Zinn, J. (1990). *Full catastrophe living: Using the wisdom of your body and mind to face stress, pain, and illness*. New York, NY: Dell.

Kaufman, G. (1989). *The psychology of shame: Theory and treatment of shame-based syndromes*. New York, NY: Springer.

Keltner, D., & Harker, L. A. (1998). The forms and functions of the nonverbal signal of shame. In P. Gilbert & B. Andrews (Eds.), *Shame: Interpersonal behavior, psychopathology and culture* (pp. 75–98). New York, NY: Oxford University Press.

Kim, S., Thibodeau, R., & Jorgensen, R. (2011). Shame, guilt, and depressive symptoms: A meta-analytic review. *Psychological Bulletin*, *137*(1), 68–96.

Kirby, J. N., & Gilbert, P. (2017). The emergence of the compassion focused therapies. In *Compassion* (pp. 258–285). London: Routledge.

Kirby, J. N., Tellegen, C. L., & Steindl, S. R. (2017). A meta-analysis of compassion-based interventions: Current state of knowledge and future directions. *Behavior Therapy*, *48*(6), 778–792.

Kupfer, D. J., Frank, E., & Phillips, M. L. (2011). Major depressive disorder: New clinical neurobiological, and treatment perspectives. *Lancet*, *20*, 1–11. doi:10.1016/50140-6736(11)60602-8

LeDoux, J. (1998). *The emotional brain*. London: Weidenfeld & Nicolson.
Lee, D. (2005). The perfect nurturer: A model to develop compassionate mind within the context of cognitive therapy. In P. Gilbert (Ed.), *Compassion: Conceptualisations, research and use in psychotherapy* (pp. 326–350). London: Routledge.
López-Castro, T., Saraiya, T., Zumberg-Smith, K., & Dambreville, N. (2019). Association between shame and posttraumatic stress disorder: A meta-analysis. *Journal of Traumatic Stress*, *32*(4), 484–495.
MacBeth, A., & Gumley, A. (2012). Exploring compassion: A meta-analysis of the association between self-compassion and psychopathology. *Clinical Psychology Review*, *32*(6), 545–552.
Maratos, F. A., Montague, J., Aziz, H., Welford, M., Wood, W., Barnes, C., . . . Gilbert, P. (2019). Compassion in the classroom: Evaluation of a compassionate mind training intervention with school staff to improve well-being. *Mindfulness*, *10*, 2245–2258. Advance Online Publication.
Maratos, F. A., Sheffield, D., Wood, W., McEwan, K., Matos, M., & Gilbert, P. (2019). *The physiological effects of a compassionate mind training course with school teachers and support staff*. Manuscript in preparation.
Matos, M. (2012). *Shame memories that shape who we are*. Doctoral Dissertation, Faculty of Psychology and Educational Sciences, University of Coimbra.
Matos, M., Albuquerque, I., Palmeira, L., Cunha, M., Lima, M. P., Maratos, F., & Gilbert, P. (2019). Building compassionate schools: Pilot study of a compassion based intervention to promote teachers' well-being, professional satisfaction and emotion regulation skills. Manuscript in preparation.
Matos, M., Carvalho, S., Cunha, M., Galhardo, A., & Sepodes, C. (2017). Psychological flexibility and self-compassion in gay and heterosexual men: How they relate to childhood memories, shame and depressive symptoms. *Journal of LGBT Issues in Counseling*, *11*(2), 88–105. Retrieved from http://dx.doi.org/10.1080/15538605.2017.1310007
Matos, M., Duarte, C., Duarte, J., Gilbert, P., & Pinto-Gouveia, J. (2018). How one experiences and embodies compassionate mind training influences its effectiveness. *Mindfulness*, *9*(4), 1224–1235. doi:10.1007/s12671-017-0864-1
Matos, M., Duarte, C., Duarte, J., Pinto-Gouveia, J., Petrocchi, N., Basran, J., & Gilbert, P. (2017). Psychological and physiological effects of compassionate mind training: A pilot randomized controlled study. *Mindfulness*, *8*(6), 1699–1712. doi:10.1007/s12671-017-0745-7
Matos, M., Duarte, J., & Pinto-Gouveia, J. (2017). The origins of fears of compassion: Shame and lack of safeness memories, fears of compassion and psychopathology. *The Journal of Psychology: Interdisciplinary and Applied*, *151*(8), 804–819. doi:10.1080/00223980.2017.1393380
Matos, M., Ferreira, C., Pinto-Gouveia, J., & Duarte, C. (2015). Eating disorders: When social ranking is shaped by early shame experiences. *Psychology and Psychotherapy: Theory, Research and Practice*, *88*(1), 38–53. doi:10.1111/papt.12027
Matos, M., & Pinto-Gouveia, J. (2010). Shame as a traumatic memory. *Clinical Psychology and Psychotherapy*, *17*, 299–312. doi:10.1002/cpp.659

Matos, M., & Pinto-Gouveia, J. (2014). Shamed by a parent or by others: The role of attachment in shame memories relation to depression. *International Journal of Psychology and Psychological Therapy, 14*(2), 217–244.

Matos, M., & Pinto-Gouveia, J. (2018a). *Shame autobiographical memory: An integrative model for the relations among autobiographical, traumatic and central shame memory features, shame feelings and psychopathology*. Submitted manuscript.

Matos, M., & Pinto-Gouveia, J. (2018b). *Understanding shame memories' phenomenology in clinical and nonclinical samples I: The shame experiences interview*. Submitted manuscript.

Matos, M., & Pinto-Gouveia, J. (2018c). *Understanding shame memories' phenomenology in clinical and nonclinical samples II: In the heat of the shame experience*. Submitted manuscript.

Matos, M., & Pinto-Gouveia, J. (2018d). *Understanding shame memories' phenomenology in clinical and nonclinical samples III: The aftermath of shame experiences*. Submitted manuscript.

Matos, M., Pinto-Gouveia, J., & Costa, V. (2013). Understanding the importance of attachment in shame traumatic memory relation to depression: The impact of emotion regulation processes. *Clinical Psychology and Psychotherapy, 20*, 149–165. doi:10.1002/cpp.786

Matos, M., Pinto-Gouveia, J., & Duarte, C. (2012). Above and beyond emotional valence: The unique contribution of the central and traumatic shame memories to psychopathology vulnerability. *Memory, 20*(5), 461–477. doi:10.1080/09658211.2012.680962

Matos, M., Pinto-Gouveia, J., & Duarte, C. (2013). Internalizing early memories of shame and lack of safeness and warmth: The mediating role of shame on depression. *Behavioural and Cognitive Psychotherapy, 41*(4), 479–493. doi:10.1017/S1352465812001099

Matos, M., Pinto-Gouveia, J., & Gilbert, P. (2013). The effect of shame and shame memories on paranoid ideation and social anxiety. *Clinical Psychology and Psychotherapy, 20*, 334–349. doi:10.1002/cpp.1766

McAdams, D. P., Josselson, R., & Lieblich, A. (Eds.). (2006). *Identity and story: Creating self in narrative*. Washington, DC: APA Books.

Mikulincer, M., & Shaver, P. R. (2004). Security-based self-representations in adulthood: Contents and processes. In W. S. Rholes & J. A. Simpson (Eds.), *Adult attachment: Theory, research, and clinical implications* (pp. 159–195). New York, NY: Guilford Press.

Miller, R., & Mason, S. E. (2005). Shame and guilt in first episode schizophrenia. *Journal of Contemporary Psychotherapy, 35*(2), 211–221.

Morrison, D., & Gilbert, P. (2001). An exploratory study of the relation between social rank, shame, and anger to provocation in primary and secondary psychopaths. *Forensic Psychiatry, 12*, 330–356.

Nathanson, D. L. (1994). *Shame and pride: Affect, sex, and the birth of the self*. New York, NY: W.W. Norton & Company.

Pace, T. W. W., Negi, L. T., Adame, D. D., Cole, S. P., Sivilli, T. I., Brown, T. D., . . . Raison, C. L. (2008). Effect of compassion meditation on neuroendocrine, innate immune and behavioral responses to psychosocial stress. *Psychoneuroendocrinology*, *34*, 87–98.

Panksepp, J. (2010). Affective neuroscience of the emotional brain mind: Evolutionary perspectives and implications for understanding depression. *Dialogues in Clinical Neuroscience*, *12*, 383–399.

Pinel, E. C. (1999). Stigma consciousness: The psychological legacy of social stereotypes. *Journal of Personality and Social Psychology*, *76*, 114–128.

Pinto-Gouveia, J., & Matos, M. (2011). Can shame memories become a key to identity? The centrality of shame memories predicts psychopathology. *Applied Cognitive Psychology*, *25*(2), 281–290. doi:10.1002/acp.1689

Rockliff, H., Karl, A., McEwan, K., Gilbert, J., Matos, M., & Gilbert, P. (2011). Effects of intranasal oxytocin on compassion focused imagery. *Emotion*, *11*(6), 1388–1396. doi:10.1037/a0023861

Rothschild, B. (2000). *The body remembers: The psychophysiology of trauma and trauma treatment*. New York, NY: W.W. Norton & Company.

Richter, A., Gilbert, P., & McEwan, K. (2010). Development of an early memories of warmth and safeness scale and its relationship to psychopathology. *Psychology & Psychotherapy: Theory, Research & Practice*, *82*, 171–184.

Rubin, D. C. (2005). Basic-systems approach to autobiographical memory. *Current Directions in Psychological Science*, *14*, 79–83.

Rubin, D. C., & Berntsen, D. (2009). The frequency of voluntary and involuntary autobiographical memories across the lifespan. *Memory & Cognition*, *37*, 679–688.

Schoenleber, M., & Berenbaum, H. (2010). Shame aversion and shame-proneness in cluster C personality disorders. *Journal of Abnormal Psychology*, *119*, 197–205.

Schore, A. N. (2001). The effects of relational trauma on right brain development, affect regulation and infant mental health. *Infant Mental Health Journal*, *22*, 201–269.

Segal, Z. V., Teasdale, J. D., & Williams, J. M. (2004). Mindfulness-based cognitive therapy: Theoretical rationale and empirical status. In S. C. Hayes, V. M. Follete, & M. M. Linehan (Eds.), *Mindfulness and acceptance* (pp. 45–65). New York, NY: Guilford Press.

Siegel, D. J. (2001). *The developing mind: How relationships and the brain interact to shape who we are*. New York, NY; London: Guilford Press.

Sommers-Spijkerman, M. P. J., Trompetter, H. R., Schreurs, K. M. G., & Bohlmeijer, E. T. (2018). Compassion-focused therapy as guided self-help for enhancing public mental health: A randomized controlled trial. *Journal of Consulting and Clinical Psychology*, *86*(2), 101.

Steindl, S. R., Buchanan, K., Goss, K., & Allan, S. (2017). Compassion focused therapy for eating disorders: A qualitative review and recommendations for further applications. *Clinical Psychologist*, *21*(2), 62–73. Retrieved from https://doi.org/10.1111/cp.12126

Steindl, S. R., Matos, M., & Creed, A. (2018). Early shame and safeness memories, and later depressive symptoms and safe affect: The mediating role of self-compassion. *Current Psychology*. Advance online publication. Retrieved from https://doi.org/10.1007/s12144-018-9990-8

Sutin, A. R., & Robins, R. W. (2008). Going forward by drawing from the past: Personal strivings, personally meaningful memories, and personality traits. *Journal of Personality*, *76*(3), 631–664. doi:10.1111/j.1467-6494.2008.00499.x

Sznycer, D., Tooby, J., Cosmides, L., Porat, R., Shalvi, S., & Halperin, E. (2016). Shame closely tracks the threat of devaluation by others, even across cultures. *Proceedings of the National Academy of Sciences*, *113*(10), 2625–2630.

Tangney, J. P. (2003). Self-relevant emotions. In M. R. Leary & J. P. Tangney (Eds.), *Handbook of self and identity* (pp. 384–400). New York, NY: Guilford Press.

Tangney, J. P., & Dearing, R. L. (2002). *Shame and guilt*. New York, NY: Guilford Press.

Taylor, S. E. (2010). Mechanisms linking early life stress to adult health outcomes. *Proceedings of the National Academy of Sciences*, *107*(19), 8507–8512.

Taylor, S. E., Eisenberger, N. I., Saxbe, D., Lehman, B. J., & Lieberman, M. D. (2006). Neural responses to emotional stimuli are associated with childhood family stress. *Biological Psychiatry*, *60*, 296–301.

Taylor, S. E., Lerner, J. S., Sage, R. M., Lehman, B. J., & Seeman, T. E. (2004). Early environment, emotions, responses to stress, and health. *Special Issue on Personality and Health: Journal of Personality*, *72*, 1365–1393.

Tracy, J. L., Robins, R. W., & Tangney, J. P. (Eds.). (2007). *The self-conscious emotions: Theory and research*. New York, NY: Guilford Press.

Tyrka, A. R., Price, L. H., Marsit, C., Walters, O. C., & Carpenter, L. L. (2012). Childhood adversity and epigenetic modulation of the leukocyte glucocorticoid receptor: Preliminary findings in healthy adults. *PLoS One*, 7(1), e30148. doi:10.1371/journal.pone.0030148

Weiss, D. S., & Marmar, C. R. (1997). The Impact of Event Scale—Revised. In J. P. Wilson & T. M. Keane (Eds.), *Assessing psychological trauma and PTSD* (pp. 399–411). New York, NY: Guilford Press.

Wheatley, J., Brewin, C., Patel, T., Hackmann, A., Wells, A., Fisher, P., & Myers, S. (2007). Imagery rescripting of intrusive sensory memories in depression. *Behaviour Therapy and Experimental Psychiatry*, *38*, 371–385.

Zessin, U., Dickhäuser, O., & Garbade, S. (2015). The relationship between self-compassion and well-being: A meta-analysis. *Applied Psychology: Health and Well-Being*, 7(3), 340–364.

# 5

# THE RISE OF MINDFULNESS AND ITS IMPACT ON MENTAL HEALTH AND WELL-BEING

*Felicia A. Huppert and Nickolas Yu*

## The context of the research

Most of us lead extremely busy lives and this can become a problem if we function mainly on autopilot, not noticing what we are experiencing. Yet being aware of our experience is fundamental to sustainable well-being and the alleviation of mental health problems. On autopilot we are likely to repeat old patterns of thinking and acting that may not serve us well.

Once we start to notice what we are experiencing, we can decide if that is really where we want to place our attention – whether it is beneficial or harmful for our well-being. Rather than being at the mercy of our busy life and our busy mind, we can learn how to choose where to place our attention. Mindfulness offers an evidence-based form of practice and training in awareness, and in how to direct attention to where we want it to be.

Mindfulness is being aware of our experience as it is happening, while maintaining an attitude of openness, interest and friendliness. The practice of mindfulness has been refined over thousands of years in a number of contemplative traditions, including several different approaches within Buddhism that developed techniques of mental training to reduce suffering and increase joy.

The rise of secular programs in the West has culminated in two carefully designed, widely used and scientifically researched programs – Mindfulness-Based Stress Reduction (MBSR) and Mindfulness-Based Cognitive Therapy (MBCT). Although there have been critiques of secular mindfulness, these are being addressed in more recent approaches (e.g. Feldman & Kuyken, 2019; Van Gordon & Shonin, 2020).

## Mindfulness processes and practice

Attention training takes the form of learning to focus on objects such as our breath, bodily sensations or sounds. Inevitably, the mind wanders and our focus is frequently interrupted by extraneous thoughts, images, emotions and sensations. In mindfulness training, the wandering mind is not seen as a failure, but as part of the practice itself – every time we notice that our mind has wandered, this provides an opportunity to refocus our attention.

Another form of attention regulation is open monitoring, where rather than focusing on a particular object, we open ourselves to whatever experiences arise. Both forms of attention regulation play an important role in our lives; focused attention is what we need when we wish to examine an object or experience in detail, while open monitoring is advantageous for exploring a novel environment or opening ourselves up to creative ideas (Lippelt, Hommel, & Colzato, 2014).

While mindfulness begins with awareness and learning to control where we place our attention, numerous other processes are involved which together confer benefits for mental health and well-being. The key processes comprise:

- Observing the experience, becoming aware and really noticing – this involves a perceptual shift, a 'stepping back' from the experience rather than being immersed in it and identifying with it. This allows us to notice how sensations, thoughts or emotions arise and drift away, which helps us to let them go rather than clinging onto them.
- Controlling where we place our attention – this allows us to choose the experiences that we wish to examine.
- Learning non-reactivity – creating space between the experience and the response to the experience. This space gives us the chance to respond more wisely, thus laying the foundations for self-regulation, including behaviour regulation and emotion regulation.

- Becoming aware of subtle sensations, thoughts and feelings – this can help us recognise emerging problematic experiences at an early stage, thereby avoiding a downward spiral. The early recognition of subtle positive experiences increases the opportunities to savour the pleasant.

In addition to describing *what we do* in mindfulness training, a very important part of the practice is *how we do it*. When we become aware of our experience, it is important that this is not done in a harsh or cold manner but with an attitude of gentle curiosity, openness, kindness and acceptance (Bishop et al., 2004). This is captured in Shapiro's term 'kind attention' and Ricard's term 'caring mindfulness.' This kindly attitude that we take towards our experience also forms the basis of self-compassion. Our inner critic may lead us to blame ourselves for our suffering, but kind compassion can replace these harsh judgements with a gentle, caring attitude to our struggles. Two of the most widely used self-compassion programs, Mindful Self-Compassion (MSC) and Compassion Focused Therapy (CFT), recognise that mindfulness is crucial to the ability to give oneself compassion. CFT emphasises the importance of patients recognising that their suffering is not their fault but is the consequence of the way evolution has shaped our brains (Gilbert, 2013). MSC emphasises our common humanity and recognises that suffering, personal failure and inadequacy are part of the shared human experience (Neff, 2003). Once we are capable of compassion towards ourselves, we become able to take steps to alleviate our own suffering.

## Underpinning research

### *Science versus hype*

Over the past two decades research and application of mindfulness training have grown exponentially. Mindfulness programs have become particularly widespread in clinical settings, in schools and in business organisations where the focus is often on mindful leadership. As with many new ideas, mindfulness has become something of a fad, and mindfulness training is being offered by people who may be ill-equipped to teach it. Being a good mindfulness trainer is not simply about conveying skills and information but also requires a deep understanding of how mental processes are experienced. Without this understanding and a personal practice, it would be difficult or impossible to impart an authentic account of the principles and practice of present moment awareness (see Crane et al., 2012). Mindfulness is probably at or near the peak of inflated expectations in the 'hype cycle' and is beginning to come under attack from detractors. The sustainability of mindfulness training as an effective evidence-based intervention requires a commitment to high-quality research, together with quality control guidelines or accreditation for mindfulness teachers.

## *Evidence for the general effects of mindfulness training on mental health and well-being*

There have been thousands of studies looking at the effects of mindfulness on reductions in symptoms of mental health conditions and increases in well-being, as well as a variety of other outcomes including cognitive function, performance and interpersonal relationships. We focus here on high quality studies that provide a clear indication of the magnitude of the mindfulness effect and the causal direction; that is, longitudinal or experimental studies that examine the effects of mindfulness training using outcome measures that can be quantified. Studies of matched groups are included where one group has undertaken mindfulness training and another serves as a control group. Even these studies have some limitations (Van Dam et al., 2018), such as the small sample size used in the majority of studies which make the findings less reliable, but the quality of mindfulness research has improved steadily over recent years. Many studies now use the gold standard methodology of a randomised controlled trial (RCT), often with an active control.

The selection of a mindfulness training (MT) program also has an influence. Some of the strongest evidence comes from standard eight-week MBSR and MBCT programs. These employ well-designed group-based curricula and use highly trained facilitators. There is also evidence of benefit from some other mindfulness programs including some specific online programs (e.g. Spijkerman, Pots, & Bohlmeijer, 2016). However, there are hundreds if not thousands of mindfulness programs that are sold as evidence-based but that have never been directly evaluated. It is all very well to develop a program that is informed by evidence of benefit from other programs, but that is no guarantee that a newly developed program will be effective.

Two recent systematic reviews which focus on studies using high quality designs have reported a range of benefits from mindfulness training (Creswell, 2017; Luberto et al., 2018). The outcome measures included both self-reports and observed behavioural outcomes such as helping behaviour in real-world and simulated settings. The results reported in these two reviews are very encouraging across numerous outcome measures, including clinical outcomes, cognitive and affective processes and interpersonal relationships, and we now summarise each of these. Specific references to these findings can be found either in these systematic reviews or in Huppert (2018).

Mindfulness training programs produce substantial benefits for patients with mental health problems, specifically depression, anxiety and substance abuse. An important study of patients with a history of recurrent depression by Kuyken et al. (2016) showed that patients were 31% less likely to have a relapse over a 60-week period compared to usual treatment, and 21% less likely compared to an active treatment group (anti-depressant medication or psycho-education). It has been suggested that mindfulness training has an additional benefit over anti-depressant medication, since medication can only facilitate changes in neural firing but not alter the structure of neural pathways, whereas mindfulness training can create or strengthen neural pathways that are conducive to healthy functioning (e.g. Rossouw, 2013). Mindfulness training can also have an indirect effect on mental health through its demonstrated benefits on physical health problems such as chronic pain and severe stress (e.g. Chiesa & Serretti, 2011; Zeidan, Grant, Brown, McHaffie, & Coghill, 2012).

Cognitive and affective processes have been shown to benefit from mindfulness training. There are improvements on problem-solving and behavioural measures of sustained attention and working memory, although the evidence does not at present support improvements in other aspects of attention such as shifting focus. Some of the strongest evidence relates to benefits on mood and emotions. Numerous studies have shown that MT increases positive affect as well as emotion regulation.

Although MT has usually focused primarily on within-person processes, there is evidence of benefit on interpersonal relationships. In a study where both members of a couple participated in a mindfulness training program, both showed significant improvement on survey and daily diary measures of levels of relationship satisfaction, autonomy, relatedness, closeness and acceptance of one another (J. W. Carson, K. M. Carson, Gil, & Baucom, 2004). The ability to take another's perspective has been shown to increase following mindfulness training (e.g. Karremans, Schellekens, & Kappen, 2016). A recent meta-analysis found mindfulness training substantially increases compassion and prosocial acts towards others even when training did not include a prosocial component (Donald et al., 2019).

The question is often asked 'How long do I need to practice each day for mindfulness to have a beneficial in effect?' Standard programs typically recommend 20–40 minutes of daily practice, but some studies have shown that as little as 10 minutes a day can produce lasting benefits (e.g. Reitz & Chaskalson, 2016). Studies specifically examining the effects of length of practice show that longer mindfulness practice can lead to greater benefits (Tang, Hölzel, & Posner, 2015).

### *Findings on the effect of mindfulness within organisations*

The overwhelming majority of studies that have examined the effects of mindfulness training in an organisational setting has been undertaken in healthcare organisations. Of these, a high proportion of studies are well-designed RCTs, although sample sizes are often quite small. This plethora of high-quality research has resulted in a number of recent systematic reviews and meta-analyses (Burton, Burgess, Dean, Koutsopoulou, & Hugh-Jones, 2017; Guillaumie, Boira, & Champagne, 2017; Spinelli, Wisener, & Khoury, 2019; van der Riet, Levett-Jones, & Aquino-Russell, 2018). They provide additional support for the benefits of mindfulness training at the individual and interpersonal level, as summarised earlier. Taken together, these reviews conclude mindfulness meditation has a positive impact on stress, anxiety, depression, burnout, sense of well-being and empathy. There are inconsistent findings in relation to very brief interventions (Gilmartin et al., 2017).

Going beyond the individual and interpersonal level, some studies have examined the relationship between mindfulness training on work performance. In a review of mindfulness and performance in the workplace, which includes many RCTs in healthcare and other organisations, Lomas et al. (2017) concludes that mindfulness has a valuable role to play in occupational contexts. However, one limitation of the reported studies is that work performance measures are all based on self-report rather than an external criterion. Several healthcare studies have included objective outcomes such as clinical errors, or patient reports of communication effectiveness or quality of care, although at the time of writing all these studies are small and mainly cross-sectional, using measures of mindfulness practise or dispositional mindfulness, rather than longitudinal studies where the effects of mindfulness training can be properly examined (Amutio-Kareaga, García-Campayo, Delgado, Hermosilla, & Martínez-Taboada, 2017). A study funded by the John Templeton Foundation used an RCT design to examine the effects of mindfulness meditation on a range of outcomes including patient reported care and communication and used social network analysis to examine whether mindfulness training among participating nurses produced a ripple effect across other members of staff. The design of this study which was led by Huppert and Atkins can be found at www.happinessandwellbeing.org/huppert. Full data analysis is currently underway.

To our knowledge there has been only one published paper to date combining an RCT design with external criterion for work performance (Reitz & Chaskalson, 2016; Reitz, Chaskalson, Olivier, & Waller, 2016). MBSR was administered to senior business leaders who underwent a customised Mindful Leader 360-degree (multi-rater) feedback. Compared to a wait-list control group, mindfulness training produced significant improvements in resilience, empathy, capacity for collaboration and the ability to lead in complex conditions as measured both by self-perception and multi-rater reports.

To date, the majority of research in mindfulness in organisations has been conducted from an individual and instrumental perspective. This narrow perspective emphasises the limits of what we can claim to know about mindfulness in organisations and it serves to highlight the issue that our knowledge is in its infancy. A seminal paper by a group of mindfulness scholars points to the importance of developing a multi-level understanding of the effects of mindfulness training within organisations, including its effects at the team level and the organisational level, using self-report and objective work-related outcomes (Rupprecht, Koole, Chaskalson, Tamdjidi, & West, 2018).

### *Effects of mindfulness training on physiology and the brain*

A systematic review and meta-analysis of randomised controlled trials found that mindfulness meditation training leads to decreased physiological markers of stress in a range of populations (Pascoe, Thompson, Jenkins, & Ski, 2017). This includes reduced systolic blood pressure and decreased heart rate although reductions on the stress hormone cortisol and some markers of immune function were variable across studies. Significant changes in cortisol levels were observed within participants but not in randomised controlled trial designs (O'Leary, O'Neill, & Dockray, 2016). An RCT that focused on responses to acute stress showed that mindfulness reduced blood pressure reactivity to acute stress exposures (Nyklíček, Van Beugen, & Van Boxtel, 2013). A systematic review that specifically examined the effects of mindfulness meditation on immune function found benefits on inflammatory markers and some but not all measures of immune function. This review also reported significant increases in telomerase activity, which is a marker of healthy biological aging (Black & Slavich, 2016).

Better regulation of the parasympathetic nervous system has also been reported following mindfulness training (Tang et al., 2009). It is likely that this effect is attributable in part to the slowing down of breathing that accompanies mindfulness practise. Slow breathing produces significant benefits on the cardiovascular, respiratory and autonomic nervous systems. Slowing down of breathing achieves a balance between sympathetic activity which is associated with arousal and parasympathetic activity which is associated with calming (Russo, Santarelli, & O'Rourke, 2017). In a number of these studies mindfulness training has been compared with standard relaxation training and MT has been shown to have effects over and above those of standard relaxation techniques (Tang et al., 2009).

Studies of brain function following mindfulness training also support the conclusion that MT does indeed have its desired effects. Compared to relaxation controls, when participants who had undergone a short period of mindfulness training were studied at rest in a brain scanner, high levels of activation occurred in areas previously shown to be involved in attention control, emotion regulation and self-awareness (Tang et al., 2015). It is interesting to ask how long it takes for changes to occur in the structure of relevant brain regions. The surprising finding is that by the end of a standard eight-week MBSR course, there are significant increases in the thickness of neuronal pathways (the brain's grey matter) in virtually all of the expected regions, including networks associated with cognitive processes (attention, learning and memory), emotion regulation, self-awareness, bodily awareness and compassion (Hölzel et al., 2011; Tang et al., 2015). A systematic review of brain changes following MBSR or MBCT found increased activity, connectivity and volume in the prefrontal cortex, the cingulate cortex, the insula and the hippocampus in stressed, anxious and healthy participants (Gotink, Meijboom, Vernooij, Smits, & Hunink, 2016).

## *Can mindfulness meditation cause harm?*

Mindfulness meditation encourages us to notice whatever we are experiencing, and our experiences may be delightful or difficult. When we are experiencing difficult thoughts, feelings or sensations we are invited to observe the experience with gentle curiosity rather than deny or avoid it. This can nevertheless produce discomfort which may be mild or severe, and could potentially cause harm without the guidance of an experienced teacher. Temporary discomfort appears to be inevitable in all forms of psychotherapy (Duggan, Parry, McMurran, Davidson, & Dennis, 2014) as participants confront distressing issues, learn new skills and apply them in painful or challenging situations.

In a comprehensive review of the few studies that report individual data in evidence-based mindfulness interventions, Baer, Crane, Miller and Kuyken (2019) report that adverse events such as worsening symptoms occur in 0–10.6% of participants. However, they are no more common in mindfulness programs than comparison conditions, are not attributable to the mindfulness program or are not clinically significant. Based on their detailed analysis, the authors offer the following perspective:

> Finally, it seems clear that many approaches to health and wellbeing can be stressful and challenging. Effective medications can have unpleasant side effects. Physical exercise can cause soreness and fatigue. Difficult experiences in meditation are sometimes seen as learning opportunities or indications of progress along the meditative path.
>
> *(p. 6)*

## *Summary of the scientific evidence*

The behavioural and neuroscience evidence converges to support the idea that mindfulness training not only reduces symptoms of mental and physical health problems, but also enhances well-being through the promotion of skills and processes that enable us to function at our best. These include the basic skills of awareness, attention and self-regulation that help us both to savour positive experiences and manage unpleasant experiences. Embedding the basic skills of noticing what we are experiencing and focussing on these experiences when we choose to, are likely to make us more successful in carrying out the tasks of our daily lives. Interpersonal relationships, including perspective taking and compassion, are also enhanced through mindfulness practice, thereby contributing to the well-being of the wider community.

## The transition from pure research to application

In the rest of this chapter we discuss the factors underlying the design, implementation and evaluation of mindfulness and compassion training in a healthcare organisation, and the implication of our findings for successful implementation in other types of organisations.

### *Program description*

The Heart of Health (HoH) Program was originally designed as a nursing and midwifery intervention within the Sydney Local Health District (SLHD), but has since been used to support other categories of healthcare staff. The program comprises two main sub-programs: Meditation-based Wellness and Compassion (MWAC) training and Positive Psychology-based Wellness and Compassion (PWAC) training. A description of the MWAC program will now be provided because mindfulness is the focus of this chapter.

### *Description of the Meditation-based Wellness and Compassion (MWAC) program*

The purpose of the MWAC program is to support staff well-being and patient and family-centred care. The vision is wise and loving care. The goals are to reduce stress and increase mindfulness, kindness, compassion, self-compassion, well-being and patient and family-centred care.

The program curriculum is organised around five core meditation practices:

1 Deep relaxation meditation (DRM) to reduce tension and stress. This practice is adapted from Bihar yoga nidra.
2 Mindfulness meditation (MM) to cultivate awareness and attention with an open, interested and friendly attitude.
3 Kindness meditation (KM) to foster well-wishing towards others.
4 Compassion meditation (CM) to promote an awareness of suffering and the willingness to prevent or alleviate it.

5 Self-compassion meditation (SCM) to learn to give ourselves as much care and compassion as we would give to someone who we deeply care for.

The program was originally developed as an ongoing series of weekly, 60-minute drop-in sessions. However, the program has since been offered in full-day workshop format. Each session was designed to include two guided meditation practices, and an exploration of key learning points. Brief discussions about a topic related to meditation are used to facilitate learning. Examples of the presentations include *Posture, Meditation safety* and *Mind wandering*. The length varies according to local context. Both the drop-in sessions and full-day workshops are face-to-face. This contact enables stronger connection and engagement, and the ability of staff to share experiences and ask questions and have real-time responses and support where required. Training is facilitated by healthcare workers from within the organisation who complete a 20-day MWAC Facilitation Development Program (FDP), and then continue their further development by participating in an ongoing MWAC Community of Practice that includes masterclasses, retreats and coaching/clinical supervision. Following the COVID-19 pandemic, the program leader Nickolas Yu identified an urgent need to support healthcare workers despite rules concerning isolation and lockdown, and has developed an online version of MWAC.

## *Evaluation of the program*

The MWAC program has been evaluated through pilot studies using a pre-post research design that included a four-month follow-up survey. The first study examined the effects of the program on participants' well-being and compassion. The participants attended the 60-minute weekly drop-in format of the MWAC. It took place in a busy emergency department and involved 85 nurses (Yu, Johnson, Nguyen, & Bowen, 2016). Participants in the second study took part in the two-day workshop format of MWAC, which investigated the impact of the program on the well-being and compassion of 35 frontline managers and clinical leaders (Yu, Fairbrother, Johnson, & Nguyen, 2017). These pilot studies have demonstrated the feasibility of the program and positive effects on well-being and compassion. In addition, a large study found that teams of nurses who had higher levels of mindfulness were less likely to make patient medication errors than teams who had lower levels of mindfulness (Wang, Welp, Ng, & Nguyen, 2020).

Further research was undertaken in collaboration with the Body, Heart and Mind in Business Research Group at University of Sydney (UoS) (to develop a measure of compassionate, patient-centred care) and with the Institute for Positive Psychology and Education at the Australian Catholic University (ACU) and UoS to investigate well-being and compassion. A grant from the John Templeton Foundation was awarded to the team to conduct an enriched RCT trial to evaluate well-being and compassion among nurses. It compared the benefits of two well-being intervention programs, one using mindfulness meditation techniques (MWAC), the other using goal-focused techniques grounded in positive psychology (PWAC). Fifty-two wards from the SLHD were randomly assigned to these two interventions or to a wait-list control group, and around 300 nurses were recruited into the study. Participants in the intervention groups received three full days of training separated by approximately one month, and were assessed at the beginning and end of the intervention period and at a five-month follow-up. One of the strengths of the study was the use of multiple methods to assess outcomes, including self-report measures, objective measures of performance, qualitative interviewing, ethnographic observation, patient reports and social network analysis to establish whether the interventions produced a ripple effect on staff who had not participated. Preliminary analysis showed a range of beneficial effects on well-being, mindfulness, compassion, self-compassion and burnout in both intervention groups, although patients reported experiencing more compassionate care from nurses in the mindfulness meditation group (Huppert, Johnson, & Atkins, 2018).

The various study results have helped inform the ongoing design and implementation of the training.

## *Strategies to consider for successful implementation*

During the project it became clear that successful implementation required a whole system approach, and recommendations related to this are shared here for those interested in developing similar programs.

### *Involving the right people from the outset*

It is important to identify a person or small group of people within the organisation who have the 'will and skill' (Landsberg, 1996) to design, implement and evaluate a mindfulness and compassion program. The 'will' needs to be characterised by a strong and long-term commitment because challenges and barriers arise, and the proper implementation and sustainability of a program does take time. Ideally, the person or small group has a heartfelt connection to mindfulness and compassion, characterised by a long-standing contemplative practice and experience working in the industry where the program is being implemented. This helps fuel the person's or group's motivation, while also having the perseverance and corporate memory to navigate the inevitable challenges and barriers that arise in organisational life.

### *Clear and compelling vision and message*

Clarifying an inspirational vision and communicating a clear and compelling message that engages the hearts and minds of people is vital. Healthcare is like many industries and organisations: fast-paced, complex, ever-changing and demanding both cognitively and emotionally. As a result, staff commonly report facing competing commitments and seemingly unending demands on their attention. With limited time and attention, it is crucial that new programs captivate the imagination and motivation of staff. Forming a simple but powerful message is therefore paramount. However doing this is not always easy because workplaces are diverse and different stakeholders find different things more or less important and attractive.

## The 'elevator pitch' for the SLHD program was:

> The vision is wise and loving care.
>
> The program exists to support staff wellness and compassionate care.
>
> When staff are happy and *well* they are more able and likely to be compassionate.
>
> Research has found that *meditation* can reduce stress, and increase well-being, mindfulness, kindness, compassion and self-compassion.
>
> MWAC is science-informed, non-religious and practical.
>
> This program is really about helping you deliver the type of care that you would want for yourself and loved ones.

Next are further messages used within SLHD to engage staff support for the program.

## Reasons to support staff wellness:

- *Work burden.* Supporting staff well-being is important because the volume, pace, complexity and emotionality of the work can take its toll on staff. The potential costs related to poor staff well-being are not just personal but also financial and social.
- *Productivity.* Staff are able to provide better patient care when they are happy and well.
- *Moral imperative.* Supporting staff wellness is a social good, in and of itself.

## Reasons to support compassionate care:

- *Patient expectations.* Patients and families don't just want care that is safe and effective, but also kind, understanding and compassionate.
- *Positive care experiences.* All healthcare organisations strive towards achieving excellence; one dimension of excellence is positive care experiences, and this includes care that is compassionate.
- *Better clinical outcomes.* Mindful and compassionate nurses are more likely to have higher quality communication and relationships with patients, and this has benefits including better information sharing, fewer patient complaints and fewer staff errors.

## Reasons to use meditation in order to support staff wellness and compassionate care:

- Meditation has been found to improve empathy, connection and compassion (Goleman & Davidson, 2017).
- Meditation has also been found to improve mental health and well-being (Creswell, 2017; Luberto et al., 2018).
- Meditation is versatile and accessible. It can be used in small and larger groups, and for brief and longer periods of time. And it can be adapted to the needs of people, including workplace applications at interpersonal, team and organisational levels (Rupprecht et al., 2018).

When delivering a message about the reason for training, it is also helpful to use narrative and creative approaches. The use of personal stories, metaphors, narratives and other creative mediums such as poetry, song, dance, art and photography can be used to stir the hearts of people. This can sometimes engage people who might not ordinarily become involved through the common means of communication in organisations.

In SLHD, the program leader (NY), used his own personal stories of caring for his parents and their experiences in hospitals. These stories were often used in important presentations, and this storytelling set the scene for a call to action. The use of story was complemented by reference to empirical research related to mindfulness, compassion and well-being. This dual strategy of using narrative and science in tandem as a call to action engaged a broader range of staff.

## *Role modelling and support by leaders throughout the organisation*

When leaders across an organisation 'walk the talk' and model mindful, compassionate behaviour, and support mindfulness and compassion in visible and ongoing ways, this sets the organisational tone and gives people permission to act in more mindful and compassionate ways.

Leaders shape an organisation in a variety of ways, including what gets talked about, when, how and how often. This means that leaders can promote mindfulness and compassion through conversational or reflective practice strategies such as mentoring, coaching, clinical supervision, journaling, action learning groups, communities of practice and staff forums. This can be a powerful strategy to help people understand, make sense of, learn from and adjust their work practices. When mindfulness and compassion are valued and prioritised in conversational and reflective spaces, then this provides valuable opportunities for staff to be mindful and compassionate.

At crucial stages of implementing mindfulness and compassion training across SLHD and beyond, two key leaders, Susan Pearce (Deputy Secretary NSW Health) and Katharine Duffy (District Director of Nursing and Midwifery), consistently encouraged staff to provide 'compassionate care, every patient, every time.' This aspirational goal was clear, compelling and challenging. Their genuine commitment provided powerful momentum for the training to be made available to staff on a wide scale. This supportive leadership has been continued by Ivanka Komunsanac (SLHD Director of Nursing). These leaders have 'walked the talk,' by taking action that has helped embed mindfulness and compassion into the workplace through the

- creation of funded wellness and compassion roles,
- enabling funding for more than 100 frontline managers and 300 clinicians to participate in full day mindfulness and compassion programs,
- formation of working groups to progress staff wellness and compassionate care,
- allocation of funding and in-kind resources to support mindfulness and compassion research, and
- continually identifying and acting on opportunities to scale and sustain the program.

Their commitment has been further demonstrated in themselves attending the program. This experiential understanding of the program has helped them be active sponsors of the program and this has set the tone for other managers to gradually see that mindfulness and compassion training is an organisational priority and is not a passing fad. This has also provided other staff with the psychological permission to support the program and attend it themselves. It is now common for managers to attend the program with clinicians. Some of these managers have now actually trained to become facilitators of the program for their staff, helping to ensure its sustainability in the local context. The commitment of health leaders such as Carolyn Rae, Steve Bernardi, Gari Chinguno, Anna Thornton, Dr. Greg Fairbrother, Dr. Teresa Anderson, Emma Brinded and Jenny Gardner has enabled the program to spread to various hospitals throughout other parts of Australia and New Zealand.

### *Gradually hardwire mindfulness and compassion into the organisation*

For training to be successful it is imperative that hardwiring takes place. Hardwiring refers to any organisational activity that helps to embed the effects of training into the workplace. SLHD has used the following hardwiring strategies: funding roles to support mindfulness and compassion; creation of funding streams to enable staff participation in training; funding for the purchase of training materials; formation of governance structures such as working groups to support mindfulness and compassion; providing resources to support research; setting key performance indicators and goals related to mindfulness and compassion; creation of strategic plans that prioritise mindfulness and compassion; running structured events like forums and conferences on mindfulness and compassion; and offering the training during work hours (thus demonstrating that self-care and compassion are core business rather than something that staff should do in their own leisure time). One of the most powerful ways that mindfulness and compassion training has been hardwired into SLHD is through the MWAC Facilitation Development Program. This in-house training of mindfulness and compassion facilitators, conducted by the author (NY), in conjunction with recognised expert meditation teachers resulted in the MWAC program being much more sustainable, scalable and cost-effective.

### *Thoughtful, deliberate and responsive strategy*

The success of a program is also shaped by the philosophical and strategic decisions that are made in the planning, implementation and evaluation of such programs. A variety of questions is worth considering in the planning stages of the program. These include, will the program be:

- Short term or run continuously?
- Implemented swiftly on a wide scale or more slowly on a smaller scale?
- Implemented in a systematic or emergent manner?
- For specific staff groups or open to all staff groups?
- Designed as a stand-alone program or integrated within a broader program?
- Remedial or universal?

The SLHD approach has been strengths-based rather than remedial. A remedial offering is characterised by beliefs such as, 'Staff are burnt-out,' and 'There is a lack of compassion in the workplace.' This has the connotation of problems, deficits and that something is wrong with people. With this approach, research and statistics are often shared with staff to demonstrate that something needs fixing. The program may then be used in organisational hotspots. This perspective can be useful in trying to get funding for programs. However, if this approach is chosen then there is the risk that some staff may react to this because they may perceive an insinuation of inadequacy or blame and as a result become angry, suspicious or resentful about the program. In contrast, a strengths-based approach emphasises gratitude for the good work that staff are already doing despite the very real challenges that they face on a daily basis as they navigate the complex, fast-paced and emotionally demanding nature of working in contemporary healthcare. SLHD's strengths-based, universal approach is informed by positive organisational scholarship and positive psychology. The key message that is shared with staff is that the program is being offered in order to support staff to continue with the great job they are already doing.

SLHD has also used a slow and small approach rather than swift and broad, where it commenced with two local nursing teams before spreading across the whole district to include all staff groups. The progressive spread of the program enabled a team of health staff within SLHD to be trained and developed as MWAC facilitators. Several cohorts of facilitators have been trained and this has gradually led to new drop-in sessions arising organically in an increasing number of work sites.

It is useful to think through who the training will be offered to first, because it is likely that training won't be able to be offered to all staff simultaneously. SLHD commenced by offering the program to nurses for three main reasons: the senior manager who sponsored the program was the chief nurse in the Sydney region; the financial support from NSW Health came through the Chief Nursing and Midwifery Office; and nurses comprise 40% of the workforce and have the most direct contact with patients. The program became so popular that other staff groups expressed interest in participating and subsequently became involved. Occasionally, the program has been implemented to support teams that had been perceived by management to be struggling in some way. Observed improvements in staff engagement and morale have helped to strengthen management support for the training.

## Other factors to consider for successful implementation

### *Anticipating and working with people's expectations about meditation*

To help people experience the benefits of mindfulness and meditation training it is important to clarify realistic expectations early on. For instance:

*Meditation isn't about being able to make the mind stop thinking* – It is more about cultivating a spacious and friendly relationship with thoughts. This is important because if people come with the expectation of 'switching off' and it doesn't happen they may believe that the practice doesn't work or that they are 'no good at it.' The reality is that minds think a lot and it can even seem that this happens more in the early days of meditation. It is possible that over time, people take their thoughts less seriously and believe that they are not their thoughts.

*Mind wandering during meditation is not failure* – Mind wandering happens a lot in life, including during meditation. With this understanding it is less likely that people will tell themselves stories such as 'I am not very good at this,' or 'See, I'm not the kind of person who can meditate.'

*We won't always feel good during meditation and this is okay* – Instead, during mindfulness meditation we are practising the ability to notice and accept whatever experiences arise, regardless of whether they are pleasant or unpleasant. Likewise, when we do heart-based practices such as kindness, compassion and self-compassion meditation, it is an act of *good will* and an expression of wanting ourselves and others to be well and free from suffering – rather than expecting ourselves to necessarily *feel good*.

*Meditation is not a panacea for all of life's conditions and problems* – People have also been exposed to overstated benefits of meditation, therefore it can be helpful for people to have a more realistic understanding of what meditation offers.

*The benefits of meditation may take time* – We live in a fast-paced society where people often expect to see results quickly. However, the benefits of meditation can be subtle and cumulative, so it can take time and practice before the results of meditation become discernible in a person's life. Helping people appreciate this means they are more likely to be patient and persevering, and as a result, meditate for long enough for meditation benefits to become more apparent.

A practical way to work with people's expectations is to ask them upfront what they hope to gain from the training and then clarify whether or not these are realistic or helpful expectations to have.

## *Meditation safety strategies*

People may resist undertaking training because they are concerned about being vulnerable and potentially overwhelmed by their own suffering or that of others. So it is important not to make people do the training. Instead a slow and gentle approach is advised. In terms of pre-existing mental illness and trauma, the potential for adverse events needs to be considered thoughtfully. People with trauma and mental illness histories should not be expected or forced to attend, particularly if they do not feel ready to. In the case that people want to it is advised they be given specific information about the contents of the training, so they can discuss this with a mental health professional in order to determine whether or not the program is a good fit for them. It is also important to consider if any modifications need to be made to meditation instructions, and that instructions are offered as an invitation rather than an expectation.

### *Concerns about mindfulness training*

Despite the potential benefits of mindfulness training, a number of criticisms about mindfulness are worth considering. First, the benefits of mindfulness may have been overinflated by some commentators. Second, mindfulness training in organisational settings has been de-contextualised from its original philosophical and ethical framework and as a result has been watered down, at times commodified, and potentially been used inappropriately. Third, mindfulness training has predominantly been used as an individual-level intervention whereas change often requires action at multiple levels including personal, organisational, social and political. Also, some people may be philosophically and spiritually opposed to mindfulness training because of its origins in Eastern philosophy. Therefore, it is important to temper any enthusiasm to implement mindfulness training into organisations, with a respectful consideration of potential concerns about the practice. Overall however, while mindfulness is not a panacea for all problems, nor is it 'everyone's cup of tea' for a variety of reasons, research evidence seems to suggest that it may benefit a broad number of people in a variety of ways.

## Lessons learnt

### *Program adaptability*

An important question to ask when introducing a mindfulness program is whether it will be implemented in a systematic manner or emergent manner. Both approaches have their advantages. Our experience in the highly demanding setting of hospital wards is that with the best will in the world, the reality is that it is not possible to stick to a highly structured and often pre-existing program and format. For instance, at a moment's notice nurses enrolled on the program can be called away to deal with urgent clinical issues. So the program format needs to be adaptable to meet these needs. In addition, as described earlier, program content should be integrated with the organisation's values, and tailored to the organisational experience of participants. We found that another important benefit of adapting the program to the context is the positive effect on participants and the organisation in being co-creators of the program.

## *Program sustainability*

A key learning was the value of embedding the program across all levels of the organisation, beginning with senior managers and leaders. This led to a sense of collaborative ownership of the program and facilitated its continued growth throughout the SLHD and beyond. The specific strategies that were adopted have been described earlier. We believe they have broad applicability to a wide range of organisations. They include the involvement of the right people from the outset, developing and communicating a clear and compelling vision and message and harnessing the support and role modelling of leaders throughout the organisation to inspire employees. The final strategy for program sustainability is to ensure that the program becomes hardwired into the organisation.

Some of the steps taken to hardwire the program into SLHD included funded roles and governance structures to support mindfulness; in-house facilitation training; and incorporating key performance indicators of mindfulness, well-being and compassion into the workplace. Equally important is committing resources to support ongoing research.

## *Program evaluation*

It is essential to continue to evaluate our programs, to ensure that they are as effective as they can be for the largest number of people, the widest range of outcomes and the longest duration of effect. We have learnt that evaluation in an unpredictable setting is not easy, and the most carefully designed research program (e.g. Huppert, Johnson, &

Atkins, 2018; www.happinessandwellbeing.org/huppert) may need to be compromised when faced with the realities of pursuing the research in contemporary, fast-paced organisations.

But this does not mean that we should put evaluation and research in the 'too hard' basket – it is too important for this. Through careful evaluation, it may be possible to tweak or refine the program in such a way that instead of showing measurable benefits on 50% of participants, it now has a positive impact on 80%. Or instead of showing benefits on a few individual or organisational outcomes, it shows benefits on a wide range of outcomes, perhaps extending its benefits to the whole of a person's life. A commitment to long-term evaluation enables us to establish whether the benefits are short-lasting or long term. It has been recognised that participants may adopt mindfulness practice as a way of life, with all the mental health and well-being benefits that it can bring, and not just a useful skill for managing stress and distress.

## *The importance of more high-quality research*

Although there is compelling evidence of the mental health and well-being benefits of mindfulness training, we are still at an early stage of our scientific understanding. For example, mindfulness training involves a number of skills and processes, and much work remains to be done to explore the relative contribution of each of these components to the overall beneficial effects on the body, mind and brain. One way to continue advancing our scientific understanding is to use well-designed, validated programs such as MBSR and MBCT which employ a carefully designed curriculum, manuals for participants and well-trained teachers. Such programs offer the consistency and replicability that is helpful in scientific research.

On the other hand, when mindfulness training is delivered in an organisation such as a school, healthcare setting or business organisation, there are advantages to adapting the program to meet the needs of the organisation.

## Concluding remarks

The diverse chapters in this book have demonstrated the effectiveness of psychological interventions to improve mental health conditions and increase well-being across the population, regardless of whether a person has a mental health condition or not. In this chapter, we make the case for mindfulness training to be regarded as one of these effective interventions. While there remains a great deal of research to be done to establish the range of mechanisms through which mindfulness practise has its benefits, we make the strong suggestion that mindfulness can be considered foundational for sustainable improvements in mental health and well-being (Huppert, 2018). We do so because mindfulness training promotes awareness of our ongoing experience and this is fundamental to learning how best to manage painful experiences or savour pleasant ones. Further, mindfulness promotes the capacity to choose where we place our attention, whether on stimuli that increase the likelihood of mental harm, or stimuli that increase the likelihood of helpful attitudes and behaviours. Awareness and attention are among the most basic of psychological processes: they underpin all other processes, so in this sense can be regarded as foundational. Mindfulness can also be regarded as foundational to compassion, since the very first step in showing compassion towards oneself and others is to be aware that suffering is being experienced. We believe the scientific evidence we have reviewed provides a compelling demonstration of the effectiveness of mindfulness training programs across a wide range of outcomes and we trust that the strategies we have outlined for implementing and embedding mindfulness programs in organisations will be of use to others embarking on this journey.

## References

Amutio-Kareaga, A., García-Campayo, J., Delgado, L., Hermosilla, D., & Martínez-Taboada, C. (2017). Improving communication between physicians and their patients through mindfulness and compassion-based strategies: A narrative review. *Journal of Clinical Medicine*, *6*(3), 33.1–17. doi:10.3390/jcm6030033

Baer, R., Crane, C., Miller, E., & Kuyken, W. (2019). Doing no harm in mindfulness-based programs: Conceptual issues and empirical findings. *Clinical Psychology Review*, *71*, 101–114. Retrieved from https://doi.org/10.1016/j.cpr.2019.01.001

Bishop, S. R., Lau, M., Shapiro, S., Carlson, L., Anderson, N. D., Carmody, J., . . . Devins, G. (2004). Mindfulness: A proposed operational definition. *Clinical Psychology: Science and Practice*, *11*(3), 230–241. Retrieved from https://doi.org/10.1093/clipsy.bph077

Black, D., & Slavich, G. (2016). Mindfulness meditation and the immune system: A systematic review of randomized controlled trials. *Annals of the New York Academy of Sciences*, *1373*(1), 13–24.

Burton, A., Burgess, C., Dean, S., Koutsopoulou, G. Z., & Hugh-Jones, S. (2017). How effective are mindfulness-based interventions for reducing stress among healthcare professionals? A systematic review and meta-analysis. *Stress and Health*, *33*(1), 3–13.

Carson, J. W., Carson, K. M., Gil, K. M., & Baucom, D. H. (2004). Mindfulness-based relationship enhancement. *Behavior Therapy*, *35*(3), 471–494.

Chiesa, A., & Serretti, A. (2011). Mindfulness-based interventions for chronic pain: A systematic review of the evidence. *The Journal of Alternative and Complementary Medicine*, *17*(1), 83–93.

Crane, R. S., Kuyken, W., Williams, J. M. G., Hastings, R. P., Cooper, L., & Fennell, M. J. (2012). Competence in teaching mindfulness-based courses: Concepts, development and assessment. *Mindfulness*, *3*(1), 76–84.

Creswell, J. D. (2017). Mindfulness interventions. *Annual Review of Psychology*, *68*, 491–516.

Donald, J. N., Sahdra, B. K., Van Zanden, B., Duineveld, J. J., Atkins, P. W., Marshall, S. L., & Ciarrochi, J. (2019). Does your mindfulness benefit others? A systematic review and meta-analysis of the link between mindfulness and prosocial behaviour. *British Journal of Psychology*, *110*(1), 101–125.

Duggan, C., Parry, G., McMurran, M., Davidson, K., & Dennis, J. (2014). The recording of adverse events from psychological treatments in clinical trials: Evidence from a review of NIHR-funded trials. *Trials*, *15*, 335.

Feldman, C., & Kuyken, W. (2019). *Mindfulness: Ancient wisdom meets modern psychology*. New York, NY: Guilford Press.

Gilbert, P. (2013). *Mindful compassion: Using the power of mindfulness and compassion to transform our lives*. London: Hachette.

Gilmartin, H., Goyal, A., Hamati, M. C., Mann, J., Saint, S., & Chopra, V. (2017). Brief mindfulness practices for healthcare providers: A systematic literature review. *The American Journal of Medicine*, *130*(10), 1219-e1.

Goleman, D., & Davidson, R. (2017). *The science of meditation: How to change your brain, mind and body*. London: Penguin.

Gotink, R. A., Meijboom, R., Vernooij, M. W., Smits, M., & Hunink, M. M. (2016). 8-Week mindfulness based stress reduction induces brain changes similar to traditional long-term meditation practice: A systematic review. *Brain and Cognition*, *108*, 32–41.

Guillaumie, L., Boira, L. O., & Champagne, J. (2017). A mixed-methods systematic review of the effects of mindfulness on nurses. *Journal of Advanced Nursing*, *73*(5), 1017–1034. doi:10.1111/jan.13176

Hölzel, B. K., Carmody, J., Vangel, M., Congleton, C., Yerramsetti, S. M., Gard, T., & Lazar, S. W. (2011). Mindfulness practice leads to increases in regional brain graymatter density. *Psychiatry Research: Neuroimaging*, *191*(1), 36–43.

Huppert, F. A. (2018). Living life well: The role of mindfulness and compassion. In *The social psychology of living well* (pp. 65–82). London: Routledge.

Huppert, F. A., Johnson, A., & Atkins, P. (2018). Towards an ideal RCT on the benefits of mindfulness: Theory versus reality in a healthcare organisation. Invited Presentation, International Conference on Mindfulness, Amsterdam.

Karremans, J. C., Schellekens, M. P. J., & Kappen, G. (2016). Bridging the sciences of mindfulness and romantic relationships: A theoretical model and research agenda. *Personality and Social Psychology Review*. doi:10.1177/1088868315615450

Kuyken, W., Warren, F. C., Taylor, R. S., Whalley, B., Crane, C., Bondolfi, G., . . . Segal, Z. (2016). Efficacy of mindfulness-based cognitive therapy in prevention of depressive relapse: An individual patient data meta-analysis from randomized trials. *JAMA Psychiatry*, *73*(6), 565–574.

Landsberg, M. (1996). *The Tao of coaching*. London: HarperCollins.

Lippelt, D. P., Hommel, B., & Colzato, L. S. (2014). Focused attention, open monitoring and loving kindness meditation: Effects on attention, conflict monitoring, and creativity – A review. *Frontiers in Psychology*, *5*, 1083.

Lomas, T., Medina, J. C., Ivtzan, I., Rupprecht, S., Hart, R., & Eiroa-Orosa, F. J. (2017). The impact of mindfulness on well-being and performance in the workplace: An inclusive systematic review of the empirical literature. *European Journal of Work and Organizational Psychology*, *26*(4), 492–513.

Luberto, C. M., Shinday, N., Song, R., Philpotts, L. L., Park, E. R., Fricchione, G. L., & Yeh, G. Y. (2018). A systematic review and meta-analysis of the effects of meditation on empathy, compassion, and prosocial behaviors. *Mindfulness*, *9*(3), 708–724.

Neff, K. D. (2003). Self-compassion: An alternative conceptualization of a healthy attitude toward oneself. *Self and Identity*, *2*(2), 85–101.

Nyklíček, I., Van Beugen, S., & Van Boxtel, G. J. (2013). Mindfulness-based stress reduction and physiological activity during acute stress: A randomized controlled trial. *Health Psychology*, *32*, 1110–1113.

O'Leary, K., O'Neill, S., & Dockray, S. (2016). A systematic review of the effects of mindfulness interventions on cortisol. *Journal of Health Psychology*, *21*(9), 2108–2121.

Pascoe, M. C., Thompson, D. R., Jenkins, Z. M., & Ski, C. F. (2017). Mindfulness mediates the physiological markers of stress: Systematic review and meta-analysis. *Journal of Psychiatric Research*, *95*, 156–178.

Reitz, M., & Chaskalson, M. (2016). Mindfulness works but only if you work at it. *Harvard Business Review Digital Articles*, 2–5.

Reitz, M., Chaskalson, M., Olivier, S., & Waller, L. (2016). *The Mindful Leader: Developing the capacity for resilience and collaboration*. Ashridge: Executive Education, Hult Research.

Rossouw, P. J. (2013). The end of the medical model? Recent findings in neuroscience regarding antidepressant medication: Implications for neuropsychotherapy. *Neuropsychotherapy in Australia*, *19*, 3–10.

Rupprecht, S., Koole, W., Chaskalson, M., Tamdjidi, C., & West, M. (2018). Running too far ahead? Towards a broader understanding of mindfulness in organisations. *Current Opinion in Psychology*, *28*, 32–36.

Russo, M. A., Santarelli, D. M., & O'Rourke, D. (2017). The physiological effects of slow breathing in the healthy human. *Breathe*, *13*(4), 298–309.

Spijkerman, M. P. J., Pots, W. T. M., & Bohlmeijer, E. T. (2016). Effectiveness of online mindfulness-based interventions in improving mental health: A review and meta-analysis of randomised controlled trials. *Clinical Psychology Review*, *45*, 102–114.

Spinelli, C., Wisener, M., & Khoury, B. (2019). Mindfulness training for healthcare professionals and trainees: A meta-analysis of randomized controlled trials. *Journal of Psychosomatic Research, 120*, 29–38.

Tang, Y.Y., Hölzel, B. K., & Posner, M. I. (2015). The neuroscience of mindfulness meditation. *Nature Reviews Neuroscience, 16*(4), 213–225.

Tang, Y. Y., Ma, Y., Fan, Y., Feng, H., Wang, J., Feng, S., . . . Zhang, Y. (2009). Central and autonomic nervous system interaction is altered by short-term meditation. *Proceedings of the National Academy of Sciences, 106*(22), 8865–8870.

Van Dam, N.T., van Vugt, M. K., Vago, D. R., Schmalzl, L., Saron, C. D., Olendzki, A., . . . Meyer, D. E. (2018). Mind the hype: A critical evaluation and prescriptive agenda for research on mindfulness and meditation. *Perspectives on Psychological Science, 13*(1), 36–61.

van der Riet, P., Levett-Jones, T., & Aquino-Russell, C. (2018). The effectiveness of mindfulness meditation for nurses and nursing students: An integrated literature review. *Nurse Education Today, 65*, 201–211.

Van Gordon, W., & Shonin, E. (2020). Second-generation mindfulness-based interventions: Toward more authentic mindfulness practice and teaching. *Mindfulness, 11*, 1–4. doi:10.1007/s12671-019-01252-1

Wang, K. L., Welp, A., Ng, J. L., & Nguyen, H. (2020). Enhancing compassion in healthcare: A multi-level perspective. In R. D. Lansbury, A. Johnson, & D. van den Broek (Eds.), *Contemporary issues in work and organisations actors and institutions*. Oxon: Routledge.

Yu, N., Fairbrother, G., Johnson, A., & Nguyen, H. (2017). Intensive meditation-based wellness and compassion training program (MWAC) yields sustained impacts among nursing and midwifery leaders at six month follow up. Presentation, Sydney Local Health District Innovation and Research Symposium, Sydney.

Yu, N., Johnson, A., Nguyen, H., & Bowen, K. (2016). Science-based, meditation program (Sankalpa) improves compassionate, patient & family-centred care: Preliminary results. Presentation, Sydney Local Health District Innovation and Research Symposium, Sydney.

Zeidan, F., Grant, J. A., Brown, C. A., McHaffie, J. G., & Coghill, R. C. (2012). Mindfulness meditation-related pain relief: Evidence for unique brain mechanisms in the regulation of pain. *Neuroscience Letters, 520*(2), 165–173.

# 6

# A NEW MODEL FOR SUSTAINABLE MENTAL HEALTH

## Integrating well-being into psychological treatment

*Ernst T. Bohlmeijer and Gerben J. Westerhof*

### Introduction

As a practising therapist or counsellor, bring to mind one of your current clients. Imagine this person as you meet him or her during your sessions together. What are the client's major complaints and problems? How does this client present him or herself? How is your client currently functioning in his or her social and societal life?

Next we would like you to imagine your client two years from now after successful treatment. What would you hope for your client? For example, how do you see the client functioning in daily life two years from now? We suppose that most therapists and counsellors will hope that their clients' complaints and problems have been resolved or have substantially diminished and they are coping well with, or adapting to, life-events, difficulties and daily hassles. But we also suppose that most of you will imagine the presence of positive functioning. Most likely you will envision your client being engaged in meaningful activities, experiencing caring and loving relationships and possibly feeling joy and happiness.

If you agree with these assumptions, you probably also agree with the idea that mental health care should not only focus on treating mental disorders and symptomatology, but also on promoting positive aspects of mental health. In this chapter, we propose a balanced perspective between a more traditional, illness-oriented approach and a broader approach that also includes well-being as an important aspect of mental health. After a brief account of the development of illness- and health-related approaches, a heuristic, balanced model of sustainable mental health is introduced that integrates dysfunctional and functional perspectives of mental health.

We will review the evidence that positive mental health can be reliably measured as well-being. We then explore the growing number of studies investigating the impact of mental well-being and its relationship with psychopathology. Sustainable mental health is realized with a spectrum of treatments and interventions targeting both dysfunctional and functional emotional, cognitive and behavioural patterns. We will discuss how a number of psychological treatments align well with a balanced focus on suffering alongside well-being. To support our thesis, we will review studies that evaluated the impact of some of these interventions on mental health. We end this chapter by outlining some challenges for the actual realization of this model of sustainable mental health.

## The need for a more balanced approach in clinical psychology

Though it seems safe to conclude that most therapists would consider indicators of positive functioning as vital outcomes of treatment, the dominant focus in measuring treatment success has been on mental disorders and symptoms of psychopathology. Maddux (2009) argued that this is due to the fact that clinical psychology adopted an illness ideology from its beginning and that, in the 20th century, clinical psychology has become increasingly illness-oriented. Terms reflect an underlying medical model such as: symptomatology, disorder, pathology, diagnosis, treatment, patient and clinician. This illness ideology can also be witnessed in ever-expanding classification instruments – such as the Diagnostic and Statistical Manual (DSM) – that have become a primary framework for treatment. Clinical psychology has become mainly concerned with what is deviant and abnormal and with maladaptive behaviours and conditions. Identifying disorders and applying interventions that aim to 'repair' underlying maladaptive functioning are considered the primary tasks of the clinician.

It is important to acknowledge that this approach has been to various degrees successful. A large body of knowledge currently exists on dysfunctional physical, neurological, psychological and social factors that cause or maintain distress and mental disorders (Davey, 2008). Evidence-based treatment guidelines and interventions for many disorders are now widely available. However, the medical model in clinical psychology has also been criticized (Gilbert, 2019; Bentall, 2010). One criticism is that the medical approach yields a tendency to over-medicalize and pathologizes various forms of suffering including those that arise from reactions to aversive life-events (Maddux, 2009). For example, shyness has gradually been transformed from being a normal behaviour into a social anxiety disorder (Lane, 2007). A second criticism is that categories of psychological disorders are socially constructed, do not represent actual discrete phenomena and, therefore, are limited in facilitating indications for specific treatments. An alternative dimensional approach to identifying individual differences in psychological phenomena such as attachment styles, emotion-regulation and cognitive patterns has been developed and is more promising in informing individualized interventions (e.g., Helzer et al., 2008; Brown & Barlow, 2005). A third criticism is that the positive dimensions of life have long been overlooked despite the fact that the question of 'what causes mental health or well-being' is equally as essential as the question concerning 'what causes mental suffering or ill-being' (Erikson, 1959; Seligman & Csikszentmihalyi, 2000). If one agrees that the presence of well-being is an important outcome in psychological interventions, then one must maintain a balanced understanding that while diminishing maladaptive functioning can reduce mental suffering, promoting adaptive functioning can yield well-being.

Many scholars have articulated this proposition over the past decades. More than 60 years ago, Marie Jahoda (1958) conducted a review of psychological theories and conceptualizations of mental health and defined six criteria of mental health, which included positive attitudes towards oneself, integration and autonomy. Building on this work, Ryff (1989) elaborated upon the concept of psychological well-being, based on a systematic review of mainly humanistic and lifespan theories on mental health and healthy human development, for example: the concept of the fully functioning person (Rogers, 1961), self-actualization (Maslow, 1954) and personal development (Erikson, 1959). Fava, Ruini, and Belaise (2007) proposed that enduring or complete recovery from mental illness should be defined as the absence of suffering and the presence of psychological well-being. In addition, he was among the first to develop a specific well-being therapy (Fava, Rafanelli, Cazzaro, Conti, & Grandi, 1998). Similarly, Keyes (2005) conceived of complete mental health as a state in which individuals are both free of psychopathology and are flourishing. Keyes (2005) defined flourishing in life as the presence of high levels of subjective well-being and positive (psychological and social) functioning. Consumers of mental health care also acknowledge the importance of well-being in recovery. In contrast to clinical recovery, personal recovery has been defined as working towards well-being, regardless of the presence of mental illness (Slade, 2010). It is a way of living a satisfying, hopeful and contributing life even within the limitations caused by illness (Anthony, 1993).

In a broader sense, positive psychology has been developed as a science of well-being and flourishing, with a focus on studying positive emotions, traits and institutions (Seligman & Csikszentmihaly, 2000). The benefits of positive psychology in the context of clinical psychology have been discussed as providing a more balanced research field, improving prediction and treatment of mental disorder and buffering negative life-events (e.g., Seligman, Rashid, & Parks, 2006; Wood & Tarrier, 2010). A growing number of studies have evaluated the impact of positive psychology interventions in clinical populations (Chakhssi, Kraiss, Sommers-Spijkerman, & Bohlmeijer, 2018). Cloninger (2006) underscored the challenge for psychiatry to improve well-being in the general population and developed an integrated psychoeducational intervention with a focus on physical, psychological and spiritual well-being. Huppert (2005) advocated population approaches to increase well-being and underscored that even small increases of well-being in the population will substantially diminish the incidence of mental illness.

Reviewing the various models of mental well-being, Vaillant (2003) distinguished six conceptual ways to assess it: 1) mental health as above normal, 2) positive psychology, 3) maturity, 4) social-emotional intelligence, 5) subjective well-being and 6) resilience. Vaillant stresses that these models complement each other and that each model describes only some aspects of mental well-being, yet often in psychology we focus on only one conceptual model as opposed to an integrative approach.

Based on this past research, we can conclude that in the last decades many appeals have been made for clinical psychology and psychiatry to broaden their scopes to include various models of mental well-being. However, we argue that no fundamental changes have evolved in clinical practice and that, despite the fact that therapists may use mental well-being theories as primary guidance for their therapies, daily clinical practice is still predominantly illness- or disorder-oriented. There is at present no systematic integration of mental well-being approaches into clinical psychology practice nor into mental health care as a whole. One reason may be that mental illness is a condition that seems to be reliably defined with clear limits while mental well-being appears to be a value judgement rather than within the domain of science (Vaillant, 2003). Whereas a humanistic approach is often difficult to reconcile with empirical evidence, positive psychology has also introduced empirical studies (Waterman, 1993). Granted, the concepts and measurements are still rather new and sometimes disputed, like the different conceptions of well-being. Another likely reason is that clinical psychologists are predominantly trained to analyze and treat symptom-defined disorders and their dysfunctional emotional, cognitive and behavioural patterns. Therefore, an orientation towards mental illness readily becomes the core DNA of their professional identity.

Given this background, we propose that the profession requires a more systematic integration of well-being into clinical psychology. Mental well-being offers new dimensions for process insights and new interventions (Vaillant, 2003). The evidence that has been lacking to support this claim is now widely available, with much more research available on positive interventions in clinical contexts (e.g., Wood & Johnson, 2016).

## Towards a model for sustainable mental health

We propose that our model of sustainable mental health provides an essential starting point for reviewing the evidence in favour of integrating positive psychology into clinical models and providing a structure to different psychological treatments. Figure 6.1 presents a heuristic model for sustainable mental health. While it is beyond the scope of this chapter to present a detailed review of the various components of the model, we will summarize the model's components next.

The first component in this model is that, in addition to reductions in symptoms of mental health difficulties and psychopathology, signs and expressions of mental well-being are seen as essential outcomes of interventions. The research we present in this chapter shows that one cannot simply assume that the absence of mental illness automatically implies the presence of well-being. Perhaps more importantly, mental well-being and mental illness are not simply each other's complement

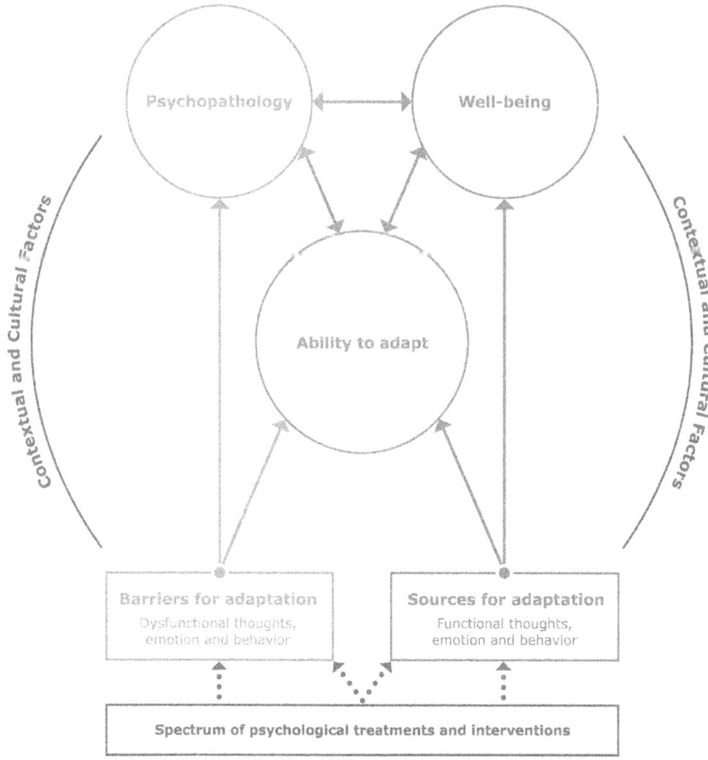


**FIGURE 6.1** Framework for sustainable mental health

and bipolar constructs, but rather hold a dynamic relationship in which both may influence the other. This is not to say that there may be times when mental illness is so dominant in people's lives that it may be difficult to imagine how well-being can also be present.

The second component of the model is the inclusion of *adaptation processes*. The absence of psychological complaints and the presence of well-being can easily be taken as normative endpoints in the sense that people are expected to strive for continuous optimal states of absence of distress or mental illness and a constant presence of mental well-being. However, it is not realistic to state that life will always be without suffering or that it will always be characterized by flourishing. We, therefore, expect that both continua of mental health will fluctuate across time. What is important to understand is how people regulate their mental well-being, particularly because such an understanding can also provide possibilities for psychological interventions. Therefore, adaptation processes appear in our model.

A third component in the model is the presence of contextual factors. Systems such as relationships, parents, organizations and communities may cause or maintain dysfunctional or maladaptive cognitions or behaviours that are related to mental illnesses or distress. However, these social and familial contexts can also enhance resources that promote adaptation and mental health. One must acknowledge that social, historical and cultural contexts play a significant role in supporting or thwarting individual attempts to maintain and achieve mental health (see also Gilbert, 1995, 2019). Although in this chapter we mainly focus on individual aspects of the model, this does not mean that individuals are solely responsible for managing their mental health. Social contexts and cultures are known to be major factors in both positive and distressing mental states (Haslam, Jetten, Cruwys, Dingle, & Haslam, 2018).

A fourth component of the model includes psychological treatments and their targets. A large number of psychological treatments have been developed in the second half of the 20th century, reflecting the growing interest in the psychological model of psychopathology. We propose that one way to categorize psychological treatments is to determine whether the treatment's primary focus for successful adaptation is targeting barriers versus resources. Currently there are no clear divisions between treatments focusing on mental illness and treatments focusing on mental well-being. Rather, psychological treatments may directly and indirectly impact both psychopathology or well-being through different underlying mechanisms.

## *Mental health and its relationship with psychopathology*

In this section, we will discuss the definition of well-being, its measurement, relationship to psychopathology and application in clinical practice.

An essential question is how to define mental health beyond the absence of illness and symptoms. The World Health Organization (WHO, 2005) defined mental health as 'a state of well-being in which the individual realizes his or her own abilities, can cope with the normal stresses of life, can work productively and fruitfully, and is able to make a contribution to his or her community' (p. 2). The three core components of this definition are 1) feeling well, 2) effective functioning of an individual and 3) effective functioning of the individual within a community.

To further operationalize these core components from the point of view of the individual's experience, Keyes (2002) drew on psychological and social research that explored the nature of well-being. Two traditions of well-being are often distinguished: hedonic well-being and eudaimonic well-being (Ryan & Deci, 2001; Waterman, 1993). Keyes (2002) equates hedonic well-being with emotional well-being. It is linked to being able to 'take pleasure from our senses', such as enjoying food, music, the smell of flowers and sex. There is now a widespread consensus that emotional well-being is a multidimensional concept, including evaluations of life in general and life domains in emotional terms (i.e., life-satisfaction) along with the presence of positive affects and the absence of negative affects (Diener, 1984; Diener, Suh, Lucas, & Smith, 1999). The concept of eudaimonia dates back to Aristotle, who believed that the essential element of a good life was the realization of one's own potential, as opposed to subjective happiness (Waterman, 1993). Ryff (1989; Ryff & Essex, 1991) has been influential in operationalizing the psychological dimension of eudaimonic well-being. He found six elements of positive functioning that make up psychological well-being: self-acceptance, purpose in life, autonomy, positive relationships with others, environmental mastery and personal growth. Each of these elements is important as one strives to realize one's potential and to live a fulfilled life. In addition to individual functioning, Keyes (1998) argued that optimal social functioning in terms of social engagement and societal functioning is also an essential aspect of eudaimonic well-being. Based on an examination of the work of classical sociologists and social psychologists, Keyes distinguished five dimensions of what he called social well-being: social coherence, social acceptance, social actualization, social contribution and social integration. Table 6.1 gives a short description of the dimensions of emotional, psychological and social well-being. In this way, mental well-being comprises the presence of both emotional well-being as an indicator of *feeling well* along with psychological and social well-being as indicators of *living well and meaningfully*. Whereas much debate about the relations and precedence of hedonic and eudaimonic well-being have ensued, Keyes (2002) considers both equally important. He defined *flourishing* as the combination of high levels of both hedonic well-being and eudaimonic well-being.

**TABLE 6.1** Short description of 14 dimensions of emotional, psychological and social well-being

| | |
|---|---|
| *Emotional well-being* | |
| Positive affect | Experiencing the presence of positive emotions and vitality. |
| Life-satisfaction | Evaluating one's life in a positive way. |
| Negative affect | Experiencing absence of severe and lasting negative emotions. |
| *Psychological well-being* | |
| Autonomy | Self-determining and independent; able to resist social pressures to think and act in certain ways; regulates behaviour from within; evaluates by personal standards. |
| Environmental mastery | Having a sense of competence in managing the environment and daily activities; able to create contexts suitable to personal needs. |
| Personal growth | Having a feeling of developing one's self and a sense of realizing one's potential; seeing improvement in one's self over time. |
| Positive relations with others | Having warm and trusting relationships with others. |
| Purpose in life | Having goals in life and a sense of direction; having meaningful goals for living. |
| Self-acceptance | Possessing a positive attitude toward oneself; acknowledging and accepting positive and negative qualities. |
| *Social well-being* | |
| Social acceptance | Having a positive attitude towards others while acknowledging people's differences. |
| Social actualization | Believing that people and society have potential and can evolve positively. |
| Social contribution | Feeling that one's life is useful to others and society. |
| Social coherence | Feeling that society and culture are intelligible and somewhat predictable and meaningful. |
| Social integration | Having a sense of belonging to a community and feeling supported by others. |

During the past decades, many reliable and valid instruments have been developed to measure well-being. The combination of the Satisfaction with Life Scale (SWLS; Pavot & Diener, 2008) and the Positive and Negative Affect Schedule (PANAS; Watson & Tellegen, 1999) is often used to assess hedonic well-being. Several instruments have been developed to assess eudaimonic aspects of well-being, but there is less consensus in this domain. Instruments that have been used are, for example, the Basic Need Satisfaction Scale that was developed from self-determination theory (Johnston & Finney, 2010) and the Flourishing Scale (Diener et al., 2009) that has a less clear theoretical foundation for its choice of items. Ryff (1989) developed the Psychological Well-Being Scales to assess psychological well-being and Keyes (1998) developed the Social Well-Being Scales to assess social well-being. A number of instruments assess aspects of both hedonic and eudaimonic well-being, and a good example is the PERMA profiler (Positive emotion, Engagement, Relationships, Meaning and Accomplishment) that is based on a positive psychological model of flourishing (Seligman, 2018).

In our own studies, we contributed to the development of the Mental Health Continuum – Short Form (MHC-SF) that was first introduced by Keyes (2005). This instrument is the only one that assesses all theoretically derived aspects of emotional, psychological and social well-being, with one item for each dimension as described in Table 6.1. The instrument was developed from longer versions of instruments that assess the three core components (Keyes, 2005). Research has consistently found support for the three-factor structure, with excellent reliability and construct validity of the Mental Health Continuum – Short Form (MHC-SF) in various healthy samples across the world, such as the United States (Robitscheck & Keyes, 2009), the Netherlands (Lamers, Westerhof, Bohlmeijer, Ten Klooster, & Keyes, 2011), South Africa (Keyes et al., 2008), Iran (Joshanloo, Wissing, Khumalo, & Lamers, 2013), North Korea (Lim, 2014) and Argentina (Perugini, De la Iglesia, Solano, & Keyes, 2017). Using advanced longitudinal Item Response Theory analyses, Lamers, Glas, Westerhof and Bohlmeijer (2012) found that the MHC-SF resulted in no differential item functioning across time, demographics and health indicators. This implies that the items are equally reliable in assessing levels of well-being across time and groups. A cross-national comparison including the Netherlands, Iran and South Africa also confirmed the measurement equivalence in different cultures (Joshanloo et al., 2013).

After defining mental well-being and providing the means to assess it, another vital question is how mental well-being relates to mental illness. There is growing evidence for the two-continua model. This model holds that mental well-being and mental illness are related yet discernible phenomena: one continuum represents the presence or absence of mental well-being, the other the presence or absence of mental illness. This two-related-factors model of mental well-being and illness has demonstrated superiority over one-factor models in large representative surveys of American, English and Dutch adults (Keyes, 2005; Lamers et al., 2011; Schotanus-Dijkstra et al., 2016; Weich et al., 2011; Westerhof & Keyes, 2010). The evidence for mental well-being and mental illness as distinct dimensions is also supported by studies examining genetics (Kendler, Myers, & Keyes, 2011), health and life-style surveys (Huppert & Whittington, 2003) and life-span studies (Westerhof & Keyes, 2010; Lamers, Glas, Westerhof, & Bohlmeijer, 2012).

Substantial longitudinal evidence indicates that higher levels of mental well-being reduce the risk of mental health problems (e.g., Grant, Guille, & Sen, 2013; Keyes, Dhingra, & Simoes, 2010; Wood & Joseph, 2010). Wood and Joseph (2010) found that people low in psychological well-being were up to seven times more likely to meet the cut-off for clinical depression ten years later. Lamers and colleagues (2015) demonstrated that three and six months later, changes in well-being were predictive of levels of psychopathology and vice versa. These bidirectional relations remained after statistically controlling for initial levels of well-being and psychopathology, revealing that both dimensions should be seen as complementary. Using data from almost 5,000 representative Dutch adults, Schotanus-Dijkstra and colleagues (2017) found that the presence of high levels of mental well-being at one moment reduced the risk of incident mood disorders by 28% and the risk of incident anxiety disorders by 53% three years later. While controlling for socio-demographics, physical health, life-events, comorbidity and clinical severity, a recent longitudinal panel study demonstrated that mental well-being positively influenced recovery from anxiety disorder three years later (Schotanus-Dijkstra, Pieterse, Drossaert, Walburg, & Bohlmeijer, 2019).

One explanation for the buffering effects of mental well-being on mental illness is that positive characteristics are helpful in successful coping/adaptation to negative life-events (Ryff, 2014; Vaillant, 2000; Wood & Tarrier, 2010). For example, the ability to experience positive emotions motivates cognitions and behaviour that promote resources for coping with future difficult life periods (Fredrickson, 1998, 2001). The adaptive and buffering effects of positive characteristics have also been demonstrated for optimism (Schiavon, Marchetti, Gurgel, Busnello, & Reppold, 2017), gratitude (Wood, Froh, & Geraghty, 2010) and positive and supportive relationships (Holeva, Tarrier, & Wells, 2001). Several reviews have also found that higher levels of mental well-being may promote recovery and reduce the risk of mortality in people with physical diseases (Chida & Steptoe, 2008; Howell, Kern, & Lyubomirsky, 2007; Lamers, Bolier, Westerhof, Smit, & Bohlmeijer, 2012).

The studies described earlier have been carried out in the general population. In more recent studies, we focused on mental well-being and illness in clinical populations. The reliability and validity of the MHC-SF were evaluated in clinical populations in a study with 472 adult psychiatric outpatients with mood, anxiety, personality, developmental and eating disorders (Franken, Lamers, Ten Klooster, Bohlmeijer, & Westerhof, 2018) and in 468 people with eating disorders (De Vos, Radstaak, Bohlmeijer, & Westerhof, 2018). Confirmatory factor analyses showed that the three-factor structure of emotional, psychological and social well-being fitted the data best. Internal consistency was high for both the total scale and the three subscales. In these studies, we also addressed the two-continua model. Again, this model had the best fit in these clinical groups, although the correlation between mental well-being and illness was substantially higher than in the general population (Franken et al., 2018; De Vos et al., 2018). Nevertheless, levels of well-being showed large variations: De Vos and colleagues (2018) found that about 26% of patients with eating disorders experienced low levels of mental well-being but another 13% experienced high levels of mental well-being. Lastly, the two-continua model has also been corroborated in outcome research. Post-hoc analyses on a large randomized controlled trial on the effects of Acceptance and Commitment Therapy (ACT) as guided self-help for depression (Fledderus, Bohlmeijer, Pieterse, & Schreurs, 2012) demonstrated that 64% of the participants receiving ACT reliably changed either their mental well-being or depression and 72% reliably changed either their mental well-being or anxiety (Trompetter, Lamers, Westerhof, Fledderus, & Bohlmeijer, 2017). This finding shows that interventions may have differential effects for mental well-being and mental illness.

All these studies support the importance of promoting mental well-being in clinical populations and the general public, as suggested by the scholars we presented in the introduction of this chapter. However, there is an additional reason why mental well-being should be integrated into clinical care: patients value mental well-being as part of their perspective on recovery. One can make a distinction between clinical and personal recovery. Whereas clinical recovery focuses on decreasing symptoms and remission, personal recovery focuses on the process that patients with mental health difficulties undergo in order to reconstruct their identity and live a meaningful life. Leamy and colleagues (2011) synthesized studies on recovery from patients' perspectives and introduced the CHIME model: Connectedness, Hope, Identity, Meaning and Empowerment. This model has close correspondence to aspects of eudaimonic well-being, and, in a recent study, it was found that there is a strong correlation between the MHC-SF and the questionnaire about the processes of recovery (QPR), a self-reporting instrument developed from the CHIME model (Kraiss et al., in revision). In a systematic review of qualitative studies on patients' perspectives of recovery among persons recovered from eating disorders, it was found that clinical indices for recovery were considered less important than aspects of recovery related to psychological well-being (De Vos & LaMarre, 2017).

### Adaptation processes

The absence of psychological complaints and the presence of well-being can easily be taken as normative endpoints in the sense that one might always strive for these optimal states of mental health. However, it is not realistic to expect that life will always be without suffering or that it will always be characterized by high levels of well-being. Therefore, we expect that both continua of mental health will fluctuate across time in a dynamic reciprocal process. Understanding how people regulate their mental health is essential, also because that understanding may provide possibilities for psychological interventions. For this reason, we have added adaptation processes to our balanced model of sustainable mental health.

Psychosocial adaptation can be seen as a *process* by which a person interacts with the psychosocial consequences of challenges in his or her life (e.g., daily hassles, chronic and/or severe physical and mental diseases, life-events such divorce, accidents and unemployment). A common view is that temporality plays a key role in adaptation (Livneh, 2001). We distinguish between short-term, intermediate and longer term adaptive challenges (see also Kashdan & Rotternberg, 2010). Short-term challenges include day-to-day events that often involve emotional reactions and expressions, such as anger, anxiety or dips in mood or confidence. These short-term reactions ask for processes of coping that mainly focus on the reduction of stress (Lazarus & Folkman, 1984). Intermediate challenges may be referred to as self-management and can include dealing with symptoms of illness, communicating with health professionals or adopting life-style changes (Barlow, Wright, Sheasby, Turner, & Hainsworth, 2002; Lorig & Holman, 2003). We can note too that there are long-term challenges that require the assimilation and accommodation of life-goals, identity and meaning in life.

A large body of psychological literature that relates to adaptation processes has focused on how to deal with stress, symptoms and illnesses. These processes are important mainly in the regulation of the illness continuum of mental health, often with a reactive focus on solving problems, restoring previous levels of functioning or bouncing back to an earlier equilibrium. Recently, positive psychology has offered a number of processes that more strongly focus on maintaining or promoting mental well-being, like paying attention to positive emotions or the use of strengths, virtues and values (Fredrickson, 2001; Lyubomirsky, Sheldon, & Schkade, 2005). Processes involved include, for example, benefit finding (Tennen & Affleck, 2005), posttraumatic growth (Tedeschi & Calhoun, 1995) and a sense of coherence (Antonovsky, 1993). These processes focus more on the maintenance of well-being, despite the presence of problems and stress, or even on growth in well-being due to stressful experiences.

In our search for adaptation processes, we were mainly looking for processes that go beyond the duality of preventing and treating mental illness or maintaining and promoting mental health. Instead, we wanted the processes to focus on maintaining a balance between an acceptance attitude towards suffering with appropriate efforts at alleviation and prevention on the one hand, and meaningful living on the other. Although many suitable concepts exist, we decided to focus on psychological flexibility and meaning-making in stories. We chose these two processes in particular because they also provide vital building blocks for the interventions we describe in the next section.

The flexibility of a system relates to its potential for change according to context. So, for example, cardiovascular sensitivity relates to the degree to which the heart can cope and adapt its responses to challenges upon it. *Psychological flexibility* is central in ACT, whose core processes of adaption are the ability to be aware of and accept one's emotions and cognitions and to commit to responding to life-situations in a way that is consistent with one's values (Hayes, 2016). The basic idea is that experiential avoidance occurs when people lose contact with negative sensations, emotions and thoughts. Trying to control such emotions is counterproductive as it leads to a reduction in behaviour and functioning and a loss of valued-based living (Hayes, Levin, Plumb-Vilardaga, Villatte, & Pistorello, 2013). Another approach is to strive for acceptance, strengthening the contact with experiences in the current moment. One process for acceptance that has captured much attention in research is mindfulness, i.e., purposeful attention to the present moment without judgement (see Chapter 5 by Felicia Huppert and Nickolas Yu in this volume). The ACT idea of psychological flexibility is to combine acceptance with commitment, i.e., to engage in behaviours that are directed towards personal values. Gilbert and Kirby (2019) also argue that acceptance must be matched with discernments for wise or moral action. Psychological flexibility has been described as a fundamental aspect of health (Kashdan & Rottenberg, 2010).

Meaning-making in stories refers to the assumption from a narrative perspective that people give meaning to themselves and their lives through stories that integrate the past, present and future (McAdams, 2006). Stories have also been described as 'selfing devices' and thus play a role in identity development at a separate level of personality. Stress, problems and life-events may result in disruption of the narrative process of meaning giving, which has also been described as narrative foreclosure (Bohlmeijer, Westerhof, Randall, Tromp, & Kenyon, 2013; Freeman, 2000). This may result in chaotic, victimic, negatively laden and meaningless stories that undermine both continua of mental health (Westerhof & Bohlmeijer, 2012). Over time, life-events may also result in a re-reading of one's life in hindsight (Randall & McKim, 2008), resulting in quest stories and perhaps the individual ultimately finding new meanings. The basic idea is that over time stress, problems and life-events may obtain new meanings that go beyond a simple dichotomy of negative or positive. This is probably most clearly found in redemption stories, which follow a typically American script (movie or book plot) in which negative events have a positive outcome (McAdams, 2006).

A systematic review has shown that the way people tell stories about themselves and their lives is related to mental health and well-being, over and beyond the Big Five personality traits (Adler, Lodi-Smith, Philippe, & Houle, 2016). These stories include affective aspects like positive affectivity or redemption motivational aspects like the fulfilment of agency and communion, as well as meaning-making processes. These meaning-making processes are related to aspects of identity development in which the way people identify with and distance themselves from difficult life experiences is key in the regulation of mental health and well-being (Westerhof & Bohlmeijer, 2012).

## *A spectrum of psychological treatments*

Keyes (2005) argued that the two-continua model may contribute to broadening and changing the goals of mental health care. Whereas mental health care has increasingly focused on the treatment and prevention of mental illness over the past decades, adding the continuum of mental well-being also opens up the potential for the protection and promotion of mental well-being.

Another component of our model of sustainable mental health includes psychological treatments and how they target mental well-being and illness. Rather than an either/or division, we propose that psychological treatments can be ordered on a spectrum, depending on whether the primary focus of treatment is targeting barriers or targeting resources for successful adaptation. Psychological treatments may, therefore, directly or indirectly impact psychopathology or well-being.

At one end of the spectrum are psychological treatments or interventions that primarily target barriers for successful adaptation, for example dysfunctional cognitions, emotion-regulation and behaviour. Cognitive behavioural therapies (CBT) may target information processing biases and negative biases in thinking such as overgeneralization and magnification or minimization, dysfunctional schema and beliefs about the world and oneself, avoidance behaviour, deficits in social skills and lack of positive events that are sources of reward or reinforcement. Psychodynamic treatments may focus on targeting dysfunctional defence mechanisms and resolving repressed conflicts and problematic relationships with attachment figures. Systemic therapies may target dysfunctional communication and support patterns in families and relationships. Medical treatments may target abnormalities in levels of brain neurotransmitters or dysfunctions of brain areas. Interpersonal therapy may target maladaptive attachment styles and metacommunication patterns.

In the past decades, many studies have been conducted to evaluate the effects of these psychological treatments for various disorders, though CBT seems to be, by far, the most evaluated treatment. Meta-analyses in general demonstrate moderate to large effects on mental illness (e.g., Cuijpers et al., 2014; Driessen et al., 2015). However, reviewing over 400 trials of psychological treatment of depression, Cuijpers (2015) concludes that the effects have probably been overestimated due to publication bias and the low quality of most studies.

At the other end of the spectrum are psychological treatments or interventions that primarily focus on developing and using resources for adaptation. Positive psychological interventions (PPIs) target positive emotions, cognitions and behaviours. Examples of PPIs are interventions to increase savoring, gratitude, optimism, the awareness and use of strengths, meaning and positive relationships. Meta-analyses have shown that it is possible to enhance emotional and psychological well-being through PPIs (Bolier et al., 2013; Sin & Lyubomirsky, 2009; Weiss, Westerhof, & Bohlmeijer, 2016). A recent meta-analysis of the effects of PPIs in clinical populations found small to moderate effects on mental well-being, depression and anxiety (Chakhssi, Kraiss, Sommers-Spijkerman, & Bohlmeijer, 2018). Some of these treatments in clinical populations are relatively new and have been studied to a much lesser extent. One example is positive psychotherapy which combines PPIs in a structured program. Small to moderate effects have been found in studies evaluating positive psychotherapy in various clinical populations (Rashid, 2015). One large study compared positive psychotherapy and CBT in women with a major depressive disorder and found no significant differences (Chaves, Lopez-Gomez, Hervas, & Vazquez, 2017). Another example is well-being therapy (WBT), a structured treatment aiming to extend periods of positive functioning and targeting the six dimensions of psychological well-being (Fava et al., 1998). WBT has been evaluated in mostly small samples of various clinical populations, yielding small to large effects on well-being (e.g., Fava, 1999; Fava et al., 2005; Ruini & Ryff, 2016).

Other psychological treatments could be placed more in the middle of the spectrum of psychological treatments, equally targeting barriers that hinder adaptation as well as resources that promote adaptation. One example is ACT. ACT has been defined as a distinctive model of behavioural and cognitive therapy with a strong focus on the context of behaviour (Hayes et al., 2013). It is partly based on a model of how language enables new forms of cognition and meaning-creation called relational frame theory. It links behavioural principles of psychological flexibility to both pathology and flourishing (Ciarrochi & Kashdan, 2013; Hayes et al., 2013). ACT targets dysfunctional patterns such as experiential avoidance while at the same time targeting resources such as awareness of and commitment to personal values. Thus, the promotion of mental well-being is a core focus in ACT (White, Gregg, Batten, Hayes, & Kasujja, 2017). Meta-analyses have found moderate effects of ACT in various clinical populations (e.g., A-Tjak et al., 2015; Veehof, Trompetter, Bohlmeijer, & Schreurs, 2016; Veehof, Oskam, Schreurs, & Bohlmeijer, 2011).

Compassion- and mindfulness-based treatments also can be placed in the middle of the treatment spectrum (e.g., Bishop et al., 2004; Gilbert, 2014; Kabat-Zinn, Massion, Kristeller, & Peterson, 1992; Neff, 2003). Although often combined, compassion and mindfulness do quite different things. Mindfulness is primarily a training in the competencies of attention and knowing awareness in different domains of functioning. Mindfulness can be focused on sensory experience (the breath sounds and sights) or what arises in the mind as it arises. See the chapter of Huppert and Yu in this book for a review of the benefits of mindfulness.

Compassion on the other hand is a motivational process that can be deliberately cultivated (Gilbert, 2014). Compassion Focused Therapy (CFT) argues that mammals, and especially humans, have evolved to be highly regulated through (caring) social relationships. There are a range of physiological systems that are specifically linked to caring and affiliative behaviour (such as aspects of the frontal cortex, the vagus nerve and hormones like oxytocin) which play fundamental roles in emotion regulation, mental health and moral behaviour (Gilbert, 2015). CFT and Compassionate Mind Training (CMT) work with clients to stimulate these care-focused motives and systems. CFT and CMT cultivate care-focused wisdom and courage to be able to work both on mental health difficulties *and* also promote stronger affiliative relations, be caring to others and generate a particular meaningful orientation to life which is to live 'to be helpful not harmful' (Gilbert, 2014, 2019). While different compassion focused models have slightly different orientations and approaches a recent meta-analysis of 21 randomised controlled trial (RCT) studies of compassion-based interventions found that they not only decrease mental health difficulties and symptoms but also improve well-being (Kirby, Tellegen, & Steindl, 2017). See the chapter by Kirby and Gilbert in this book for an elaborate description of compassion and compassion focused therapy.

Another approach which can also be placed in the middle of the spectrum is life-review. Life-review interventions focus on the integration of both positive and negative memories across one's whole lifespan (Westerhof, 2019). There is considerable evidence that life-review results in moderate decreases in depressive symptoms as well as in moderate increases in different aspects of well-being and positive functioning (Bohlmeijer, Smit, & Cuijpers, 2003; Bohlmeijer, Roemer, Smit, & Cuijpers, 2007; Pinquart & Forstmeier, 2012). The strongest effects are found for clinical populations and are similar to those of cognitive behavioural therapy in older adults (Pinquart & Forstmeier, 2012). A number of studies have shown that increases in meaning in life mediate the effects of life-review interventions on depressive symptoms thereby providing evidence for the working mechanism of life-review interventions (Korte, Cappeliez, Bohlmeijer, & Westerhof, 2012; Lamers, Westerhof, Glas, & Bohlmeijer, 2015; Reker, Birren, & Svensson, 2012; Westerhof, Bohlmeijer, Pot, & Beljou, 2010).

## Implementation and evidence of impact

At the Centre for eHealth and Well-Being Research at the University of Twente in the Netherlands, we have been working on several projects to corroborate and implement the model for sustainable mental health.

Our first line of research has been to include the MHC-SF in large panel studies in the general Dutch population alongside the instruments used to assess psychopathology and mental illness (e.g., Lamers et al., 2015; Schotanus-Dijkstra et al., 2016). We presented the results of these studies in the first sections of this chapter. In combination with other international studies, there is now a body of knowledge supporting the notion that mental health difficulties and mental well-being are two related but distinct phenomena and that the presence of mental well-being reduces the risk of mental illness occurring. This line of research increasingly shows the health gains that can be reached at a population level by focusing on both continua.

There has been some criticism of the model. For example, the instruments used for assessing mental health difficulties (the Brief Symptom Inventory; BSI) and the MHC-SF have slightly different answering formats: the BSI asks for the intensity of feelings during the past week, and the MHC-SF asks for the frequency of feelings during the past month. In our pilot study of a representative Dutch panel, we addressed this issue and compared the correlation of the original versions of the BSI and the MHC-SF to the correlation where the answering format of the MHC-SF was similar to that of the BSI. The correlation for emotional, social and psychological well-being for the similar format ($r = -.53, -.41$ and $-.42$; $n = 151$) was stronger than for the different format ($r = -.46, -.21$ and $-.25$; $n = 145$), but not significantly so.

A second line of research has been to collaborate closely with mental health care institutes. Several institutes have implemented the MHC-SF in their routine outcome monitoring system. As we have discussed, the first studies have demonstrated that in people with mental illnesses the correlation between mental illness and mental well-being is stronger than in the general population, but the two-continua model still holds as superior to a one-dimensional model (De Vos et al., 2018; Franken et al., 2018). A substantial percentage of persons with various mental illnesses are still able to maintain adequate levels of well-being or even to flourish despite their mental health problems (De Vos et al., 2018; Franken et al., 2018). These cross-sectional studies were based on assessments at the start of psychological treatment. As assessments of mental health and psychopathology are conducted at a regular basis during psychological treatment, in the near future, we will be able to study longitudinal relationships between mental well-being and mental illness.

Two interesting issues have emerged during this project, possibly hindering the enduring implementation of the MHC-SF as an outcome measure in mental health care. First, despite the excellent reliability of the MHC-SF in the context of research, clients find some of the MHC-SF questions difficult to answer. For example, some people find it difficult to rate the exact frequency in time or to understand the rather abstract items on social well-being. We have, therefore, simplified the answer format and some of the items on social well-being. We are currently evaluating the psychometric properties of this more practice-friendly version of the MHC-SF. Second, both clients and therapists have indicated that they do not understand the rationale of the MHC-SF in the context of treatment, undermining the motivation to fill out the questionnaire and use the results as guidance for the focus of the therapy. Such queries have exposed the need for both professionals and clients to be informed about the relevance of mental health in the context of treatment. We are now developing a guide for therapists about mental health and the MHC-SF. This guide will include a framework on how to interpret the scores on the questionnaire, how therapists can discuss the results with their clients and possible interventions to increase mental well-being. We have also developed a leaflet for clients with information about mental well-being, complete recovery and the MHC-SF. The next step will be to organize meetings in mental health care institutes and during conferences to inform professionals about these new developments.

A third line of research has been to develop new interventions that align well with the model of sustainable mental health and to evaluate the impact of these interventions in the context of public mental health promotion and psychological treatment. Given the high prevalence of common mental disorders such as depression and anxiety, there is need for early, low-intensity interventions. (Guided) self-help inventions are promising in this respect, as research has shown them to be as effective as face-to-face treatments (Cuijpers, Donker, van Straten, & Andersson, 2010; Van het Hof, Cuijpers, & Stein, 2009).

In one project a self-help book for depression was developed based on ACT and mindfulness: *Beginners Guide of Mindfulness* (Bohlmeijer & Hulsbergen, 2017). The first part of the book has readers reflect on their avoidance and control strategies and whether these strategies are effective in the long term. In the second part, readers learn how to come into contact with their current difficult experiences without trying to avoid or control them. The capacity to defuse from cognitions is amply practised. The third part focuses on building a courageous willingness to live a life that is consistent with one's personal values and to experience a sense of purpose and meaning that these values bring. In addition, manuals for implementing the *Beginners Guide of Mindfulness* as a group course and as guided self-help were developed. Significant moderate to large effects on depression, well-being and psychological flexibility and mindfulness were found in various large trials that compared intervention in a group format and intervention as guided self-help to waiting-list control groups (Bohlmeijer, Fledderus, Rokx, & Pieterse, 2011; Bohlmeijer, Lamers, & Fledderus, 2015; Fledderus et al., 2012). *Beginners Guide of Mindfulness* has also been implemented as an eHealth intervention and similar effects were found (Pots et al., 2016). The effects were maintained at six and 12 months, thereby demonstrating a sustained impact on distress and well-being. A trial is being conducted evaluating the effectiveness of *Beginners Guide of Mindfulness* as guided self-help for older adults with anxiety symptoms (Witlox, Kraaij, Bohlmeijer, & Spinhoven, 2018). The program is now widely implemented in mental health care and financed by some major insurance companies in the Netherlands.

In a similar vein, a self-help program covering eight modules based on positive psychotherapy was developed (Schotanus-Dijkstra, Drossaert et al., 2017). Each module consists of psychoeducation and evidence-based positive psychology exercises concerning six key components of mental health: positive emotions, discovering and using strengths, optimism and hope, self-compassion, resilience and positive relations (Bohlmeijer & Hulsbergen, 2018). Adults with low to moderate levels of well-being were invited to participate in a pragmatic trial and randomly assigned to positive psychotherapy as guided self-help or to a waiting list. Moderate to large effects on mental health and distress were found up to 12 months after baseline for those participants in the self-help program (Schotanus-Dijkstra, Drossaert et al., 2017), again suggesting a sustained impact on public mental health. Increases in positive relationships and self-compassion were found to be the strongest mediators of the effects on mental health and distress (Schotanus-Dijkstra et al., 2019).

In other studies, we evaluated the impact of compassionate mind training for adults with suboptimal well-being or mild distress (Sommers-Spijkerman, Trompetter, Schreurs, & Bohlmeijer, 2018a). Adults with a low to moderate level of well-being were recruited in the general Dutch population and randomized to compassionate mind training as guided self-help ($n$ = 121) or a waitlist control group ($n$ = 122). Participants completed measures of well-being and psychological distress at baseline, post-intervention (three months) and three- and nine-month follow-up. The primary outcome was well-being, assessed with the MHC-SF. Secondary outcomes were depressive and anxiety symptoms, stress, self-compassion, self-criticism, self-reassurance, positive and negative affect, and gratitude. Compared to the waitlist control group, the compassion training group showed superior improvement on well-being and all secondary outcomes at post-intervention and three-month follow-up. In addition, the effects of the compassionate mind training were found to be mediated by self-reassurance and self-criticism (Sommers-Spijkerman, Trompetter, Schreurs, & Bohlmeijer, 2018b).

We also assessed interventions based on life-review for older adults with moderate depressive symptoms (Korte, Bohlmeijer, Westerhof, Cappeliez, & Smit, 2012; Westerhof, Lamers, Postel, & Bohlmeijer, 2019), in particular with a focus on the retrieval of specific positive memories across one's lifespan (Westerhof, Bohlmeijer, & McAdams, 2017).

Collectively these intervention studies demonstrate that early interventions based on psychological treatments that fit well with the model for sustainable mental health can have a substantial and sustained impact on mental well-being and mental illness. Furthermore, these effects are at least partially mediated by increases in the ability to adapt (psychological flexibility) and positive resources (positive relationships, self-compassion, mindfulness, positive emotions and meaning in life).

A fourth line of research has focused on psychological treatments for people with more severe mental health problems through the implementation of interventions that promote mental well-being and help to develop adaptive resources. The model for sustainable mental health allows the design of various treatment pathways. One obvious flow of treatment is to start by focusing on managing mental illness symptoms and then to shift to a mental well-being perspective. As an example of this pathway, we adapted well-being therapy (WBT; Meulenbeek, Christenhusz, & Bohlmeijer, 2015) as a rehabilitation therapy for patients who have responded to an evidence-based treatment for posttraumatic stress disorder (PTSD) and compared it to treatment-as-usual (TAU; Radstaak, Huning & Bohlmeijer, 2020). WBT was found to be more effective than TAU for participants with low levels of well-being at baseline. The effects were large for well-being and posttraumatic growth at nine months follow-up. These findings suggest that WBT can be effective in the rehabilitation of patients with PTSD when levels of well-being are still low after psychological treatment that targets symptoms of PTSD.

In a current project, we are evaluating a new eight-week group intervention, Living Well with Bipolar Disorder, for people with bipolar disorder in remission (Kraiss, Ten Klooster, Crispijn, Kupka, & Bohlmeijer, 2018). The intervention aims to improve personal recovery and well-being. The intervention comprises evidence-based positive psychology and compassion exercises (Schotanus-Dijkstra, Drossaert et al., 2017; Spijkerman-Sommers, Trompetter, Schreurs, & Bohlmeijer, 2018). Core themes are self-compassion and common humanity, compassionate balancing emotion-systems, positive emotions and dampening, coping with fear of relapse, personal goals and strengths, and positive relationships (Kraiss et al., 2018). This intervention is being compared to care-as-usual, and the primary outcomes being evaluated are well-being and personal recovery. Various reviews have underscored the potential benefits of positive psychology interventions for people with mental illnesses (e.g., Chakhssi et al., 2018; Rashid, 2015; Weiss et al., 2016).

Another research project that we are currently working on is the development of a narrative intervention for people with personality disorders (Westerhof et al., 2017). The goal of this intervention is to support people with personality disorders in their personal and social recovery. People write and share stories in a triptych: stories about the past that they want to carry along with them in their recovery trajectory; stories about choices, turning points or trajectories that made them decide to search for help; and stories about their expectations for the future after treatment has finished. These stories are collected into a printed book with help of a digital platform. We developed this intervention by combining the best available evidence on life story interventions, the expertise of clinicians and the preferences and values of people with personality disorders themselves. Its feasibility is currently being evaluated. Similar projects have addressed the effectiveness of narrative interventions for persons with psychiatric problems and intellectual disability (Westerhof, Beernink-Wassink, & Sools, 2016) as well as for persons with dementia (Elfrink, Zuidema, Kunz, & Westerhof, 2017).

These studies show that interventions focusing on both barriers to and resources for adaptation can be fruitful for people who suffer from more severe mental illnesses. An immediate challenge is to determine how to best combine these well-being interventions with more traditional approaches and to determine when exactly to offer each type of intervention during the course of treatment. We have now mainly focused on implementation towards the end of traditional treatment in order to strengthen recovery and prevent relapse. Another possibility would be to start with a number of sessions promoting resources for adaptation, such as compassion, positive emotions or positive relationships, and then implement a treatment targeting symptoms of mental illness. The assumption would be that clients who have more resources for adaptation and mental health would benefit to a great extent from intensive and confronting treatments (Trompetter, Bohlmeijer, Lamers, & Schreurs, 2016). Alternatively, one could systematically integrate positive interventions into existing treatment protocols for mental illness.

## Conclusion: directions for future innovation and research

The call for a broader approach to mental health has existed for decades. Although the implementation of such an approach has lagged behind more traditional treatments, the time is ripe for a more balanced psychological treatment that might yield sustainable mental health. We have tried to contribute to this vision by developing a theoretical model of sustainable mental health, instruments to assess mental well-being and interventions to support adaptation. We believe that enhancing positive functioning has great potential for improving the prevention and treatment of mental illness and promoting mental well-being and the ability to adapt. The presence of mental well-being as a core outcome of mental health care will make the impact of psychological treatments on clinical and personal recovery more sustainable. The model presented in this chapter aims to integrate perspectives on dysfunctional and adaptive functioning and thereby surpasses a simplistic distinction between 'negative' versus 'positive' psychology. We have discussed a selection of the growing evidence that corroborates a model of sustainable mental health and the need for more balanced psychological treatments.

However, some challenges for the actual implementation of sustainable mental health care still exist. One such challenge is that contemporary clinical psychology prioritizes a conception of human beings that is largely based on pathology and dysfunctionality. This illness-orientation has been dominant in research and education from the beginnings of psychology as a scientific and professional discipline (Maddux, 2009), and, consequentially, it may be difficult for professionals to imagine it otherwise. We foresee at least two ways in which this may change in the near future. The first is to implement the science of well-being and positive psychology into mainstream psychology and clinical psychology educational programs. At our university, we developed a master program that uses the model of sustainable mental health as the main framework for its learning objectives. The students learn to classify disorders, to assess factors that cause and maintain symptoms of mental illness and to apply the basics of cognitive behavioural therapy. But they also learn to assess emotional and psychological well-being and to apply positive psychology interventions. Additionally, we are witnessing mental health care institutes' growing interest in positive psychology and the implementation of treatments based on well-being therapy and positive psychotherapy. Increasingly, mental health care professionals are augmenting their treatments to include ACT, compassion based and narrative interventions that integrate perspectives on positive functioning and flourishing. The second development that will facilitate implementing the model of sustainable mental health and a more balanced treatment is the growing interest in personal recovery. The voice of mental health care users is becoming stronger, and their needs will have a rising impact on the development of innovative services. Public interest is rising for treatments that promote the ability to live a joyful, meaningful and engaged life, even in the presence of mental illness symptoms (e.g., Kraiss et al., 2018; Slade, 2010).

Another major challenge is to develop and implement interventions that are tailored to the needs of people across cultures and education levels. In some of the studies we presented in this chapter, the majority of the participants were Caucasian and higher educated, limiting the generalizability of the findings (e.g., Schotanus-Dijkstra, Drossaert et al., 2017). It has been found that this population is overly represented worldwide in studies on positive psychology interventions (Hendriks et al., 2018). However, some interventions may already be highly adaptive to various cultures. Life-story interventions focus on personal memories that are related to specific cultural contexts. The emphasis in ACT on clarification of personal values boosts its cross-cultural applicability (White et al., 2017). The exploration of values 'allows a natural cultural adaptation that is sensitive to the individual and yet maintains contact with underlying behavioral processes' (Hayes, Muto, & Masuda, 2011, p. 236).

Despite the remaining challenges facing the integration of well-being into psychological treatment both in practice and research, the science of mental well-being has the potential to increase the impact of psychological treatments and population approaches in the context of public mental health. Integrating mental well-being as a core outcome of psychological treatment and implementing interventions that promote positive behaviour, emotions and cognitions can yield a more balanced perspective and approach and promises to create a more sustained impact on mental health.

## References


Adler, J. M., Lodi-Smith, J., Philippe, F. L., & Houle, I. (2016). The incremental validity of narrative identity in predicting well-being: A review of the field and recommendations for the future. *Personality and Social Psychology Review, 20*, 142–175.

Anthony, W. A. (1993). Recovery from mental illness: The guiding vision of the mental health system in the 1990s. *Innovations and Research, 2*, 17–24.

Antonovsky, A. (1993). The structure and properties of the sense of coherence scale. *Social Science and Medicine, 36*, 725–733.

A-Tjak, J. G. L., Davis, M. L., Morina, N., Powers, M. B., Smits, J. A. J., & Emmelkamp, P. M. G. (2015). A meta-analysis of the efficacy of Acceptance and Commitment Therapy for clinically relevant mental and physical health problems. *Psychotherapy and Psychosomatics, 84*, 30–36.

Barlow, J., Wright, C., Sheasby, J., Turner, A., & Hainsworth, J. (2002). Self-management approaches for people with chronic conditions: A review. *Patient Education Counseling, 48*, 177–187.

Bentall, R. P. (2010). *Doctoring the mind: Why psychiatric treatments fail*. London: Penguin.

Bishop, S. R., Lau, M., Shapiro, S., Carlson, L., Anderson, N. C., & Carmody, J. (2004). Mindfulness: A proposed operational definition. *Clinical Psychology: Science and Practice, 11*, 230–241.

Bohlmeijer, E. T., Fledderus, M., Rokx, A., & Pieterse, M. (2011). The effects of ACT as an early intervention for adults with psychological distress, results of a randomized controlled trial. *Behaviour Research Therapy, 49*, 62–67.

Bohlmeijer, E. T., & Hulsbergen, M. L. (2017). *Beginners guide to mindfulness*. London: McGraw-Hill.

Bohlmeijer, E. T., & Hulsbergen, M. L. (2018). *Using positive psychology everyday: Learn how to flourish*. London: Routledge.

Bohlmeijer, E. T., Lamers, S. M. A., & Fledderus, M. (2015). Flourishing in people with depressive symptomatology increases with Acceptance and Commitment Therapy: Post-hoc analyses of a randomized controlled trial. *Behaviour Research and Therapy, 65*, 101–106.

Bohlmeijer, E. T., Roemer, M., Smit, F., & Cuijpers, P. (2007). The effects of life-review on life-satisfaction and well-being: Results of a meta-analysis. *Aging & Mental Health, 11*, 291–300.

Bohlmeijer, E. T., Smit, F., & Cuijpers, P. (2003). Effects of reminiscence and life-review on late-life depression: A meta-analysis. *International Journal of Geriatric Studies, 18*, 1088–1094.

Bohlmeijer, E. T., Westerhof, G. J., Randall, W., Tromp, T., & Kenyon, G. (2013). Narrative foreclosure in later life, preliminary considerations of a new sensitizing concept. *Journal of Aging Studies, 25*, 364–370.

Bolier, L., Haverman, M., Westerhof, G. J., Riper, H., Smit, F., & Bohlmeijer, E. T. (2013). Positive psychology interventions: A meta-analysis of randomized controlled studies. *BMC Public Health, 13*, 119.

Brown, T. A., & Barlow, D. H. (2005). Dimensional versus categorical classification of mental disorders in the 5th edition of the DSM and beyond: Comment on the special section. *Journal of Abnormal Psychology, 114*, 551–556.

Chakhssi, F., Kraiss, J. T., Sommers-Spijkerman, M., & Bohlmeijer, E. T. (2018). The effects of positive psychology interventions on well-being and distress in clinical samples with psychiatric or somatic disorders: A systematic review and meta-analysis. *BMC Psychiatry, 18*, 211.

Chaves, C., Lopez-Gomez, I., Hervas, G., & Vazquez, C. (2017). A comparative study on the efficacy of a positive psychology intervention and a cognitive behavioral therapy for clinical depression. *Cognitive Therapy and Research, 41*, 417–433.

Chida, Y., & Steptoe, A. (2008). Positive psychological well-being and mortality: A quantitative review of prospective observational studies. *Psychosomatic Medicine, 70*, 741–756.

Ciarrochi, J., & Kashdan, T. B. (2013). The foundations of flourishing. In T. B. Kashdan & J. Ciarrochi (Eds.), *Mindfulness, acceptance and positive psychology* (pp. 1–29). Oakland, CA: New Harbinger Press.

Cloninger, C. R. (2006). The science of well-being: An integrated approach to mental health and its disorders. *World Psychiatry, 5*, 2.

Cuijpers, P. (2015). Psychotherapies for adult depression: Recent development. *Current Opinions in Psychiatry*, *28*, 24–29.

Cuijpers, P., Donker, T., van Straten, A., & Andersson, G. (2010). Is guided self-help as effective as face-to-face psychotherapy for depression and anxiety disorders? A systematic review and meta-analysis of comparative outcome studies. *Psychological Medicine*, *40*, 1943–1957.

Cuijpers, P., Karyotake, E., Weitz, E., Andersson, G., Hollon, S. D., & van Straten, A. (2014). The effects of psychotherapies for major depression in adults remission, recovery and improvement: A meta-analysis. *Journal of Affective Disorders*, *159*, 118–126.

Davey, G. (2008). *Psychopathology, research, assessment and treatment in clinical psychology*. Oxford: BPS Blackwell.

De Vos, J. A., & LaMarre, A. (2017). Identifying fundamental criteria for eating disorder recovery: A systematic review and qualitative meta-analysis. *Journal of Eating Disorders*, *5*, 34.

De Vos, J. A., Radstaak, M., Bohlmeijer, E. T., & Westerhof, G. J. (2018). Having an eating disorder and still being able to flourish? Examination of pathological symptoms and well-being as two continua of mental health in a clinical sample. *Frontiers in Psychology*, *9*, 2145.

Diener, E. (1984). Subjective well-being. *Psychological Bulletin*, *95*, 542–575.

Diener, E., Suh, E. M., Lucas, R., & Smith, H. L. (1999). Subjective well-being: Three decades of progress. *Psychological Bulletin*, *125*, 276–302.

Diener, E., Wirtz, D., Tov, W., Kim-Prieto, C., Choi, D., Oishi, S., & Biswas-Diener, R. (2009). New well-being measures: Short scales to assess flourishing and positive and negative feelings. *Social Indicators Research*, *97*, 143–156.

Driessen, E., Hegelmaier, L. M., Abbass, A. A., Barber, J. P., Dekker, J. J. M., Van Henricus, L., . . . Cuijpers, P. (2015). The efficacy of short-term psychodynamic psychotherapy for depression: A meta-analytic update. *Clinical Psychology Review*, *42*, 1–15.

Elfrink, T. R., Zuidema, S. U., Kunz, M., & Westerhof, G. J. (2017). The effectiveness of creating an Online Life Story Book on persons with early dementia and their informal caregivers: A protocol of a randomized controlled trial. *BMC Geriatrics*, *17*, 95.

Erikson, E. H. (1959). *Identity and the life cycle*. New York, NY: International Universities Press.

Fava, G. A. (1999). Well-being therapy: Conceptual and technical issues. *Psychotherapy and Psychosomatics*, *68*, 171–179.

Fava, G. A., Rafanelli, C., Cazzaro, M., Conti, S., & Grandi, S. (1998). Well-being therapy: A novel psychotherapeutic approach for residual symptoms of affective disorders. *Psychological Medicine*, *28*, 475–480.

Fava, G. A., Ruini, C., & Belaise, C. (2007). The concept of recovery in major depression. *Psychological Medicine*, *37*, 307–317.

Fava, G. A., Ruini, C., Rafanelli, C., Finos, L., Salmaso, L., Magnelli, L., & Siriqatti, S. (2005). Well-being therapy of generalized anxiety disorder. *Psychotherapy and Psychosomatics*, *74*, 26–30.

Fledderus, M., Bohlmeijer, E. T., Pieterse, M. E., & Schreurs, K. G. M. (2012). Acceptance and Commitment Therapy as guided self-help for psychological distress and positive mental health: A randomized controlled trial. *Psychological Medicine*, *42*, 485–495.

Franken, C. P. M., Lamers, S. M. A., Ten Klooster, P. M., Bohlmeijer, E. T., & Westerhof, G. J. (2018). Validation of the Mental Health Continuum-Short Form and the dual continua model of well-being and psychopathology in an adult mental health setting. *Journal of Clinical Psychology*, *74*, 2187–2202.

Fredrickson, B. (1998). What good are positive emotions? *Review of General Psychology*, *2*, 300–319.

Fredrickson, B. (2001). The role of positive emotions in positive psychology: The broaden-and-build theory of positive emotions. *American Psychologist*, *56*, 218–226.

Freeman, M. (2000). When the story's over: Narrative foreclosure and the possibility of self-renewal. In M. Andrews, S. D. Sclater, & C. Squire (Eds.), *Lines of narrative: Psychosocial perspectives* (pp. 81–91). New York, NY: Routledge.

Gilbert, P. (1995). Biopsychosocial approaches and evolutionary theory as aids to integration in clinical psychology and psychotherapy. *Clinical Psychology and Psychotherapy*, *2*, 135–156.

Gilbert, P. (2014). The origins and nature of compassion focused therapy. *British Journal of Clinical Psychology*, *53*, 6–41.

Gilbert, P. (2015). Affiliative and prosocial motives and emotions in mental health. *Dialogues in Clinical Neuroscience*, *17*, 381–389.

Gilbert, P. (2019). Psychotherapy for the 21st century: An integrative, evolutionary, contextual, biopsychosocial approach. *Psychology and Psychotherapy Special Edition: Building an Integrative Science for Psychotherapy for the 21st-Century*, *92*, 164–189.

Gilbert, P., & Kirby, J. N. (2019). Preface and Introduction: Challenges of building an integrative science for psychotherapy for the 21st-century. *Psychology and Psychotherapy Special Edition: Building an Integrative Science for Psychotherapy for the 21st-Century*, *92*, 151–163.

Grant, F., Guille, C., & Sen, S. (2013). Well-being and the risk of depression under stress. *PloS One*, *8*, e67395.

Haslam, C., Jetten, J., Cruwys, T., Dingle, G. A., & Haslam, A. S. (2018). *The new psychology of health: unlocking the social cure*. London: Routledge.

Hayes, S. C. (2016). Acceptance and commitment therapy, relational frame theory and the third wave of behavioral and cognitive therapies, republished article. *Behavior Therapy*, *47*, 869–885.

Hayes, S. C., Levin, M. E., Plumb-Vilardaga, J., Villatte, J. L., & Pistorello, J. (2013). Acceptance and commitment therapy and contextual behavioral science: The progress of a distinctive model of behavioral and cognitive therapy. *Behavior Therapy*, *44*, 180–198.

Hayes, S. C., Muto, T., & Masuda, A. (2011). Seeking cultural competence from the ground up. *Clinical Psychology: Science and Practice*, *18*, 232–237.

Helzer, J. E., Kraemer, H. C., Krueger, R. F., Wittchen, H., Sirovatka, P. J., & Regier, D. A. (2008). *Dimensional approaches in diagnostic classification: Refining the research agenda for DSM-V*. Arlington, VA: American Psychiatric Association.

Hendriks, T., Warren, M. A., Schotanus-Dijkstra, M., Hassankhan, A., Graafsma, T., Bohlmeijer, E. T., & Jong, J. de. (2018). How weird are positive psychology interventions? A bibliometric analysis of randomized controlled trials on the science of well-being. *Journal of Positive Psychology*. Retrieved from doi.org/10.1080/17439760.2018.1484941

Holeva, V., Tarrier, N., & Wells, A. (2001). Prevalence and predictors of acute stress disorder and PTSD following road traffic accidents: Thought control strategies and social support. *Behavior Therapy*, *32*, 65–83.

Howell, R. T., Kern, M. L., & Lyubomirsky, S. (2007). Health benefits: Meta-analytically determining the impact of well-being on objective health outcomes. *Health Psychology Review*, *1*, 83–136.

Huppert, F. A. (2005). Positive mental health in individuals and populations. In F. A. Huppert, N. Baylis, & B. Keverne (Eds.), *The science of well-being* (pp. 307–342). Oxford: Oxford University Press.

Huppert, F. A., & Whittington, J. E. (2003). Evidence for the independence of positive and negative well-being: Implications for quality of life assessment. *British Journal of Health Psychology*, *8*, 107–122.

Jahoda, M. (1958). *Current concepts of positive mental health*. New York, NY: Basic Books.

Johnston, M. M., & Finney, S. J. (2010). Measuring basic needs satisfaction: Evaluating previous research and conducting new psychometric evaluations of the basic needs satisfaction in general scale. *Contemporary Educational Psychology*, *35*(4), 280–296.

Joshanloo, M., Wissing, M. P., Khumalo, I. P., & Lamers, S. M. A. (2013). Measurement invariance of the Mental Health Continuum-Short Form (MHC-SF) across three cultural groups. *Personality and Individual Differences*, *55*, 755–759.

Kabat-Zinn, J., Massion, A. O., Kristeller, J., & Peterson, L. G. (1992). Effectiveness of a meditation-based stress reduction program in the treatment of anxiety disorders. *American Journal of Psychiatry*, *149*, 936–943.

Kashdan, T. B., & Rottenberg, J. (2010). Psychological flexibility as a fundamental aspect of health. *Clinical Psychology Review*, *30*, 865–878.

Kendler, K. S., Myers, J. M., & Keyes, C. L. M. (2011). The relationship between the genetic and environmental influences on common externalizing psychopathology and mental wellbeing: twin research. *Twin Research Human Genetics*, *14*, 516–523.

Keyes, C. L. M. (1998). Social well–being. *Social Psychology Quarterly*, *61*, 121–140.

Keyes, C. L. M. (2002). The mental health continuum: From languishing to flourishing in life. *Journal of Health and Social Behavior*, *43*, 207–222.

Keyes, C. L. M. (2005). Mental illness and/or mental health? Investigating axioms of the complete state model of health. *Journal of Consulting and Clinical Psychology*, *73*, 539–548.

Keyes, C. L. M., Dhingra, S. S., & Simoes, E. J. (2010). Change in level of positive mental health as a predictor of future risk of mental illness. *American Journal of Public Health*, *100*, 2366–2371.

Keyes, C. L. M., Wissing, M. P., Potgieter, J. P., Temane, M., Kruger, A., & van Rooy, S. (2008). Evaluation of the Mental Health Continuum – Short Form (MHC – SF) in Setswana-speaking South Africans. *Clinical Psychology and Psychotherapy*, *15*, 181–192.

Kirby, J. N., Tellegen, C. L., & Steindl, S. R. (2017). A meta-analysis of compassion-based interventions: Current state of knowledge and future directions. *Behavior Therapy*, *48*(6), 778–792. doi:10.1016/j.beth.2017.06.003

Korte, J., Bohlmeijer, E. T., Westerhof, G. J., Cappeliez, P., & Smit, F. (2012). Life-review therapy for older adults with depressive symptomatology: Evaluation in a pragmatic randomized controlled trial. *Psychological Medicine*, *42*, 1163–1173.

Korte, J., Cappeliez, P., Bohlmeijer, E. T., & Westerhof, G. J. (2012). Meaning in life and mastery mediate the relationship of negative reminiscence with psychological distress among older adults with mild to moderate depressive symptoms. *European Journal of Ageing*, *9*, 343–351.

Kraiss, J. T., Ten Klooster, P. M., Crispijn, M., Kupka, R., & Bohlmeijer, E. T. (2018). B-positive: A randomized controlled trial of a multicomponent positive psychology intervention for euthymic patients with bipolar disorder – study protocol and intervention development. *BMC Psychiatry*, *18*, 335.

Kraiss, J. T., Ten Klooster, P. M., Crispijn, M., Kupka, R., & Bohlmeijer, E. T. (in revision). Measuring personal recovery in people with bipolar disorder and exploring its relationship with well-being and social-role participation. *Psychotherapy and Psychosomatics*.

Lamers, S. M. A., Bohlmeijer, E. T., Korte, J., & Westerhof, G. J. (2015). The efficacy of life-review as online-guided self-help for adults: A randomized trial. *The Journals of Gerontology Series B: Psychological Sciences and Social Sciences*, *70*, 24–34.

Lamers, S. M. A., Bolier, L., Westerhof, G. J., Smit, F., & Bohlmeijer, E. T. (2012). The impact of emotional well-being on long-term recovery and survival in physical illness: A meta-analysis. *Journal of Behavioral Medicine*, *35*, 538–547.

Lamers, S. M. A., Glas, C. A. W., Westerhof, G. J., & Bohlmeijer, E. T. (2012). Longitudinal evaluation of the Mental Health Continuum- Short Form (MHC-SF). *European Journal of Psychological Assessment*, *28*, 290–296.

Lamers, S. M. A., Westerhof, G. J., Bohlmeijer, E. T., Ten Klooster, P. M., & Keyes, C. L. M. (2011). Evaluating the psychometric properties of the Mental Health Continuum-Short Form (MHC-SF) in the Dutch population. *Journal of Clinical Psychology*, *67*, 99–110.

Lamers, S. M. A., Westerhof, G. J., Glas, C. A. W., & Bohlmeijer, E. T. (2015). The bidirectional relation between positive mental health and psychopathology in a longitudinal representative panel study. *The Journal of Positive Psychology*, *6*, 553–560.

Lane, C. (2007). *Shyness: How normal behavior became a sickness*. New Haven, CT: Yale University Press.

Lazarus, R. S., & Folkman, S. (1984). *Stress, appraisal and coping*. New York, NY: Springer.

Leamy, M., Bird, V., Le Boutillier, C., Williams, J., & Slade, M. (2011). Conceptual framework for personal recovery in mental health: Systematic review and narrative synthesis. *The British Journal of Psychiatry*, *199*, 445–452.

Lim, Y.-J. (2014). Psychometric characteristics of the Korean Mental Health Continuum–Short Form in an adolescent sample. *Journal of Psychoeducational Assessment*, *32*, 356–364.

Livneh, H. (2001). Psychological adaptation to chronic illness and disability: A conceptual framework. *RCB*, *44*, 151–160.

Loriq, K. R., & Holman, H. (2003). Self-management education: History, definition, outcomes, and mechanisms. *Annual Behavioral Medicine*, *26*, 1–7.

Lyubomirsky, S., Sheldon, K., & Schkade, D. (2005). Pursuing happiness: The architecture of sustainable change. *Review of General Psychology*, *9*, 111–131.

Maddux, J. (2009). Stopping the 'madness': Positive psychology and deconstructing the illness ideology and the DSM. In S. J. Lopez & C. R. Snyder (Eds.), *Oxford handbook of positive psychology* (2nd ed., pp. 61–69). New York, NY: Oxford University Press.

Maslow, A. H. (1954). *Motivation and personality*. London: Harper & Row Publishers.

McAdams, D. (2006). *The redemptive self: Stories Americans live by*. New York, NY: Oxford University Press.

Meulenbeek, P., Christenhusz, L., & Bohlmeijer, E.T. (2015). Well-being therapy in the Netherlands; letter to the editor. *Psychotherapy and Psychosomatics*, *84*, 316–317.

Neff, K. (2003). Self-compassion: An alternative conceptualization of a healthy attitude toward oneself. *Self and Identity*, *2*, 85–101.

Pavot, W., & Diener, E. (2008). The satisfaction with life scale and the emerging construct of life satisfaction. *Journal of Positive Psychology*, *3*, 137–152.

Perugini, M. L., de la Iglesia, G., Castro Solano, A., & Keyes, C. L. (2017). The Mental Health Continuum-Short Form (MHC-SF) in the Argentinean context: Confirmatory factor analysis and measurement invariance. *European Journal of Psychology*, *3*, 93–108.

Pinquart, M., & Forstmeier, S. (2012). Effects of reminiscence interventions on psychosocial outcomes: A meta-analysis. *Aging & Mental Health*, *16*, 541–558.

Pots, W. T. M., Fledderus, M., Meulenbeek, P. A. M., Ten Klooster, P. M., Schreurs, K. M. G., & Bohlmeijer, E. T. (2016). Acceptance and commitment therapy as a web-based intervention for depressive symptoms: Randomised controlled trial. *British Journal of Psychiatry*, *208*, 69–77.

Radstaak, M., Huning, L., & Bohlmeijer, E. T. (2020). Well-being therapy as rehabilitation therapy for patients with PTSD-symptoms: A randomized controlled trial. *Journal of Traumatic Stress*. Retrieved from doi.org/10.1002/jts22500

Randall, W., & McKim, E. (2008). *Reading our lives: The poetics of growing old*. New York, NY: Oxford University Press.

Rashid, T. (2015). Positive psychotherapy: A strength-based approach. *The Journal of Positive Psychology, 10*, 25–40.

Reker, G. T., Birren, J. E., & Svensson, C. M. (2012). Restoring, maintaining, and enhancing personal meaning in life through autobiographical methods. In P. T. P. Wong (Ed.), *The human quest for meaning: Theories, research, and applications* (2nd ed., pp. 383–407). New York, NY: Routledge/Taylor & Francis Group.

Robitschek, C., & Keyes, C. L. M. (2009). Keyes's model of mental health with personal growth initiative as a parsimonious predictor. *Journal of Counseling Psychology, 56*, 321–329.

Rogers, C. R. (1961). *On becoming a person*. London: Constable & Robinson Ltd.

Ruini, C., & Ryff, C. D. (2016). Using eudaimonic well-being to improve lives. In A. M. Wood & J. Johnson (Eds.), *The Wiley handbook of positive clinical psychology* (pp. 153–166). Hoboken, NJ: Wiley Blackwell.

Ryan, R. M., & Deci, E. L. (2001). On happiness and human potentials: A review of research on hedonic and eudaimonic well-being. *Annual Review of Psychology, 52*, 141–166.

Ryff, C. D. (1989). Happiness is everything, or is it? Explorations on the meaning of psychological well-being. *Journal of Personality and Social Psychology, 57*, 1069–1081.

Ryff, C. D. (2014). Psychological well-being revisited: Advances in the science and practice of eudaimonia. *Psychotherapy and Psychosomatics, 83*, 10–28.

Ryff, C. D., & Essex, M. J. (1991). Psychological well-being in adulthood and old age: Descriptive markers and explanatory processes. *Annual Review of Gerontology and Geriatrics, 10*, 144–171.

Schiavon, C. C., Marchetti, E., Gurgel, L. G., Busnello, F. M., & Reppold, C. T. (2017). Optimism and hope in chronic disease: A systematic review. *Frontiers in Psychology*, 7, 2022.

Schotanus-Dijkstra, M., Drossaert, C. H. C., Pieterse, M. E., Boon, B., Walburg, J. A., & Bohlmeijer, E. T. (2017). An early intervention to promote well-being and flourishing and reduce anxiety and depression: A randomized controlled trial. *Internet Interventions, 9*, 15–24.

Schotanus-Dijkstra, M., Pieterse, M. E., Drossaert, C. H. C., Walburg, J. A., & Bohlmeijer, E. T. (2019). Possible mechanisms in a multicomponent email guided positive psychology intervention to improve mental well-being, anxiety and depression: A multiple mediation model. *The Journal of Positive Psychology, 14*, 141–155.

Schotanus-Dijkstra, M., Pieterse, M. E., Drossaert, C. H. C., Westerhof, G. J., de Graaf, R., ten Have, M., . . . Bohlmeijer, E. T. (2016). What factors are associated with flourishing? Results from a large representative national sample. *Journal of Happiness Studies, 17*, 1351–1370.

Schotanus-Dijkstra, M., Ten Have, M., Lamers, S. M. A., De Graaf, R., & Bohlmeijer, E. T. (2017). The longitudinal relationship between flourishing mental health and incident mood, anxiety and substance use disorders. *European Journal of Public Health*, *27*, 563–568.

Seligman, M. (2018). Perma and the building blocks of well-being. *The Journal of Positive Psychology*, *13*, 333–335.

Seligman, M., & Csikszentmihalyi, M. (2000). Positive psychology: An introduction. *American Psychologist*, *55*, 5–14.

Seligman, M., Rashid, T., & Parks, A. (2006). Positive psychotherapy. *American Psychologist*, *61*, 774–788.

Sin, N. L., & Lyubomirsky, S. (2009). Enhancing well-being and alleviating depressive symptoms with positive psychology interventions: A practice-friendly meta-analysis. *Journal of Clinical Psychology*, *65*, 467–487.

Slade, M. (2010). Mental illness and well-being: The central importance of positive psychology and recovery approaches. *BMC Health Services Research*, *10*, 26.

Sommers-Spijkerman, M. P. J., Trompetter, H. R., Schreurs, K. M. G., & Bohlmeijer, E. T. (2018a). Compassion-focused therapy as guided self-help for enhancing public mental health: A randomized controlled trial. *Journal of Consulting and Clinical Psychology*, *86*, 101–115.

Sommers-Spijkerman, M., Trompetter, H. R., Schreurs, K. M. G., & Bohlmeijer, E. T. (2018b). Pathways to improving mental health in compassion-focused therapy: Self-reassurance, self-criticism and affect as mediators of change. *Frontiers in Psychology*, *9*, 2442.

Tedeschi, R. G., & Calhoun, L. G. (1995). *Trauma and transformation: Growing in the aftermath of suffering*. Thousand Oaks, CA: Sage.

Tennen, H., & Affleck, G. (2005). Benefit finding and benefit-reminding. In C. R. Snyder & S. J. Lopez (Eds.), *Handbook of positive psychology* (pp. 584–597). New York, NY: Oxford University Press.

Trompetter, H. R., Bohlmeijer, E. T., Lamers, S. M. A., & Schreurs, K. M. G. (2016). Positive psychological wellbeing is required for online self-help acceptance and commitment therapy for chronic pain to be effective. *Frontiers in Psychology*, 7, 353.

Trompetter, H. R., Lamers, S. M. A., Westerhof, G. J., Fledderus, M., & Bohlmeijer, E. T. (2017). Both positive mental health and psychopathology should be monitored in psychotherapy: Confirmation for the dual-factor model in acceptance and commitment therapy. *Behaviour Research and Therapy*, *91*, 58–63.

Vaillant, G. (2000). Adaptive mental mechanisms: Their role in a positive psychology. *American Psychologist*, *55*, 89–98.

Vaillant, G. (2003). Mental health. *American Journal of Psychiatry*, *160*, 1373–1384.

Van het Hof, E., Cuijpers, C., & Stein, D. J. (2009). Self-help and internet-guided interventions in depression and anxiety disorders: A systematic review of meta-analyses. *CNS Spectr*, *14*, 34–40.

Veehof, M. M., Oskam, M. J., Schreurs, K. M. G., & Bohlmeijer, E. T. (2011). Acceptance-based interventions for the treatment of chronic pain: A systematic review and meta-analysis. *Pain*, *152*, 533–542.

Veehof, M. M., Trompetter, H. R., Bohlmeijer, E. T., & Schreurs, K. M. G. (2016). Acceptance- and mindfulness-based interventions for the treatment of chronic pain: A meta-analytic review. *Cognitive Behaviour Therapy*, *45*, 5–31.

Waterman, A. (1993). Two conceptions of happiness: Contrasts of personal expressiveness (eudaimonia) and hedonic enjoyment. *Journal of Personality and Social Psychology*, *64*, 678–691.

Watson, D., & Tellegen, A. (1999). Issues in the dimensional structure of affect: Effects of descriptors, measurement error, and response formats. *Psychological Bulletin*, *125*, 601–610.

Weich, S., Brugha, T., King, M., McManus, S., Bebbington, P., Jenkins, R., . . . Stewart-Brown, S. (2011). Mental well-being and mental illness: Findings from the Adult Psychiatric Morbidity Survey for England 2007. *The British Journal of Psychiatry*, *199*, 23–28.

Weiss, L. A., Westerhof, G. J., & Bohlmeijer, E. T. (2016). Can we increase psychological well-being? The effects of interventions on psychological well-being: A meta-analysis of randomized controlled trials. *PLoS One*, *11*, e0158092.

Westerhof, G. J. (2019). Life review: Lifespan development, meaning processes, and interventions. In F. Gibson (Ed.), *International perspectives on reminiscence, life review and life story work* (pp. 312–326). London: Jessica Kingsley.

Westerhof, G. J., Beernink-Wassink, J., & Sools, A. M. (2016). Who am I? A life story intervention for persons with intellectual disability and psychiatric problems. *Intellectual and Developmental Disabilities*, *54*, 173–186.

Westerhof, G. J., & Bohlmeijer, E. T. (2012). Life stories and mental health: The role of identification processes in theory and interventions. *Narrative Works: Issues, Investigations & Interventions*, *2*, 107–128.

Westerhof, G. J., Bohlmeijer, E. T., & McAdams, D. P. (2017). The relation of ego integrity and despair to personality traits and mental health. *The Journals of Gerontology: Series B*, *72*, 400–407.

Westerhof, G. J., Bohlmeijer, E. T., Pot, A. M., & Beljou, I. van. (2010). The effects of the reminiscence program 'in search of meaning' on the experience of personal meaning in life: A randomized clinical trial. *The Gerontologist*, *50*, 541–549.

Westerhof, G. J., & Keyes, C. L. M. (2010). Mental illness and mental health: The two continua model across the lifespan. *Journal of Adult Development*, *17*, 110–119.

Westerhof, G. J., Lamers, S. M. A., Postel, M. G., & Bohlmeijer, E. T. (2019). Online therapy for depressive symptoms: An evaluation of counselor-led and peer-supported life review therapy. *The Gerontologist*, *59*, 135–146.

White, R. G., Gregg, J., Batten, S., Hayes, L. L., & Kasujja, R. (2017). Contextual behavioral science and global mental health: Synergies and opportunities. *Journal of Contextual Behavioral Science*, *6*, 245–251.

Witlox, M., Kraaij, V., Bohlmeijer, E. T., & Spinhoven, P. (2018). An internet-based Acceptance and Commitment Therapy intervention for older adults with anxiety complaints: Study protocol for a cluster randomized controlled trial. *Trials*, *19*, 502.

Wood, A. M., Froh, J. J., & Geraghty, A. W. A. (2010). Gratitude and well-being: A review and theoretical integration. *Clinical Psychological Review, 30.*
Wood, A. M., & Johnson, J. (2016). *The Wiley handbook of positive clinical psychology*. Hoboken, NJ: Wiley Blackwell.
Wood, A. M., & Joseph, S. (2010). The absence of positive psychological (eudemonic) well-being as a risk factor for depression: A ten year cohort study. *Journal of Affective Disorders, 122*, 213–217.
Wood, A. M., & Tarrier, N. (2010). Positive clinical psychology: A new vision and strategy for research and practice. *Clinical Psychology Review, 30*, 819–829.
World Health Organization. (2005). *Promoting mental health: Concepts, emerging evidence, practice*. Geneva: WHO.

# INDEX

Note: Page numbers in *italics* indicate a figure and page numbers in **bold** indicate a table on the corresponding page.